WHAT PEOPLE ARE SAYING ABOUT
HOLISTIC COUNSELING

In combining mind-body medicine and psychology in a nature-cure naturopathic medicine context, *Holistic Counseling* offers much needed practical tools and perspectives for physicians and patients alike, bringing the roots of natural healing to life. Dr. Moshe is a pioneering, true naturopathic physician, honoring and following in the footsteps of his ancestors and beyond, even expanding the essential teachings. This book both remains true to long expressed core traditional naturopathic principles and philosophy and at the same time presents practically applied and integrated powerful and effective healing therapeutics. With this book, Dr. Moshe would make our founders proud and will make all naturopathic physicians, other health-care practitioners and their patients filled with gratitude as they use his guidance to support getting well, healing, and curing.

Dr. Paul Epstein, ND

This book is a must for my practice book collection. Holistic Counseling has been a true blessing for my patients and for me as a Naturopathic Physician. Thank you Dr. Moshe for your hard work and dedication to your craft.

Dr. Sandra Jones, ND, LAc

Holistic Counseling − Introducing "The Vis Dialogue" is an incredibly insightful, masterful and majestic piece of work. Dr. Moshe's understanding and teaching of wholeness and healing chronic illness should be part of every Holistic institution's curriculum. As a Naturopathic Physician, I have used HC with amazing, life-changing results. There is nothing more powerful and sustaining than one's own self-discovery of the cause of their illness as it lives within them. I would highly recommend this book along with the Holistic Counseling training to anyone who has a true healer's desire to restore the sick to health.

Dr. Ron Matthias, ND, MTN Medical Group, Scottsdale, AZ

Dr. Moshe has poured his heart, experience, knowledge and truth into this book which is so important for the naturopathic community as it so eloquently explains THE root cause. There are a few reasons why I had to read *Holistic Counseling – Introducing "The Vis Dialogue"* slowly. I was reveling in the truth of each sentence, as there are so many and so profound! This book engages the reader in a dialogue for self-healing. "Reader heal thyself." No reader will walk away without having related their experience to the amazing case examples in the book, thereby engaging in self-healing. I've had breakthroughs by asking myself the same questions, and by realizing our collective experiences. While sometimes our intention as healers is to relieve our patients from their suffering, this book asks us to pause, dig deeper and to touch the wound of the person in front of us, in order for true healing to occur. As a healer, the book outlines a simple yet deep philosophical framework for counseling others. While simple in theory, it is ground-breaking and very much needed today. Profound points are made easy to grasp with clear examples and patient cases.

Vanessa Jane Ruiz, RN, BSN, Doctor of Naturopathic Medicine Candidate, 2016

Holistic Counseling has drastically changed my understanding of disease and approach to healing. I strongly believe that Holistic Counseling should be taught in all Naturopathic medical schools, as it gives students and doctors the tools necessary to address the mind-emotion-body connection at the deepest level. It is now undeniable to me how our false beliefs and emotions affect our physiology. This book is a pivotal resource to all physicians serious about helping their patients truly heal.

Dr. Caitlin Barbiero, ND

A truly outstanding perspective on the Healing Power of Nature. In *Holistic-Counseling – Introducing "The Vis Dialogue,"* Dr. Moshe took the best of psychology and holistic medicine and created one of the most powerful strategies for healing. The patient will no longer put the responsibility of their health in the hands of the physician, as with this therapy the patient will quickly realize that the fate of their health resides solely within them.

Dr. Carlye Luft, NMD

If it is possible for a book to be deeply and astoundingly profound, yet simultaneously pragmatic and beneficial in its practicality, Dr. Moshe's book, *Holistic-Counseling – Introducing "The Vis Dialogue"* succeeds admirably. Focusing on practicing true "holism" of the mind, emotions, and body, *Holistic-Counseling – Introducing "The Vis Dialogue"* is a desperately needed resource for Holistic practitioners in our day. Challenging practitioners to return to an authentic, holistic model, Dr. Moshe does not leave us with a merely theoretical book. He masterfully explains what a holistic counseling model truly entails in the first part of the book, then, as if taking us by the hand, he leads us into the second section with detailed instruction and examples of the holistic counseling method. Full of wisdom, compassion, and exemplary instruction, *Holistic-Counseling* is destined to refocus and reshape our current trends in Holistic Medical Practice.

Teresa Glick, Traditional Naturopath

This book is awesome. In this important compendium for Holistic and Naturopathic medicine, Dr. Block takes his readers on a fascinating journey from ancient philosophy to modern medicine to describe his simple yet powerful counseling technique. This enlightening book, along with the HC course, is an ideal complement for a professional health practitioner seeking deeper healing for their patients and themselves.

Dr. Erin Moore, ND

In *Holistic Counseling – Introducing "The Vis Dialogue"*, Dr. Block suggests a revolutionary way to view your patient as more than just a cluster of symptoms and how to treat them through the practice of Holistic Counseling, as opposed to the all too commonly used Allopathic Model. If more practitioners from the Western Model, Naturopathic Model and any other vein of client care would take the time to read this book and use Holistic Counseling in their practice, our patients and clients would be given the opportunity to truly heal as opposed to simply having their symptoms masked. We owe it to ourselves to live in true alignment with our soul's journey in this life and to help our patients achieve the same, all in the name of optimal health and a loving life!

Laura Henry, BScPN, RPN

As difficult as the task is of defining the mind-body connection, Dr. Moshe delivers simply and effectively. His gentle direct, yet subtle questioning produces the most profound aha moments imaginable. This book will create long overdue new and amazing paradigm shifts in the world of Holistic Medicine, in its focus on the root cause. Bravo Dr. Moshe!

Gayle C. Russell – Life Coach

In *Holistic Counseling – Introducing "The Vis Dialogue,"* Dr. Moshe passes on his masterful technique of drawing the sub-conscious into awareness, bringing out the story beneath the story. Those students who practice it diligently will find themselves equipped to lead others into deep and profound healing. Holistic Counseling should be read and studied by all those in the healing profession.

Micah McLaughlin, Naturopathic Practitioner and Founder of Continuum Healing, Grand Rapids, MI

Dr. Moshe Daniel Block is a wonderful teacher and has developed a wonderful tool for assisting patients. I'm so glad that he has put his work in a book to share with other practitioners.

Dr. Monique Aucoin, ND

After taking the Holistic Counseling class and reading this book, I can say with conviction that what Dr. Moshe teaches in this book is extremely powerful and absolutely life-changing! What I learned from Dr. Moshe was far more valuable to me than what I learned during my four years in undergrad studying for my B.S. in Psychology. After Holistic Counseling, I was able to tear down the cobwebs and find the hidden issues that I had been dealing with. Once I realized the power that I had given to my false beliefs, I was able to defeat them. Because the root issues are now gone, I have truly been able to know and understand myself more and heal on the deepest level (physician heal thyself). Now, I have the ultimate tool in my "physician's tool belt" to share with others and help them to their own self-healing! I truly enjoyed reading this and getting a "refresher course"!

Brittany M. Bennett, Doctor of Naturopathic Medicine Candidate 2018

Holistic Counseling - Introducing "The Vis Dialogue" is an essential manual for any holistic practitioner and can be easily applied into practice. Dr. Moshe Block has created an effective framework for "going down the rabbit hole" into a person's psyche, guiding the person to arrive at their OWN truth about their suffering which is integral for true healing to take place.

Dr. Olivia Greenspan, Registered Nurse, ND

Dr. Moshe takes one through the past paradigms of thought and medicine to bring you to understanding the next shift towards holism in health, living, and consciousness. Combining the study of numerous sources of medicine and through the observations one can make of Nature, he helps one to learn deep secrets of life that often are only attributed to the sages of history. *The Vis Dialogue* shows how complex we are as humans and how subtle we can create disharmony, but also correct it in our lives and for our health. I believe this book contains the answers many are looking for. More importantly, this book can be the manual for the practitioner or the individual to start asking themselves the right questions that lead to healing in profound and miraculous ways.

Dr. Bryce Healy, ND, theholistic-solution.com

This book is a testament to the inner truth we all desire to unlock within ourselves. Dr. Moshe has shown me how to embrace my fears, share my hardships, and welcome a brighter future now that I have accepted the great challenge of living on Earth. He will open your mind to the thought patterns that are not self-serving, and bring you to a higher sense of existence. His knowledge has allowed me to grow by leaps and bounds in a short period of time. I cannot thank him enough.

Dr. Cory Ostroot, ND

Testimonials of Students and Doctors that have taken Holistic Counseling – the Course

One of the best experiences of my young medical career and quite frankly, my life.

Michael J. McPherson, ND candidate, President of the NatPath Society, SCNM

Dr. Moshe's holistic counselling course provided me with such a broadened understanding of the mental-emotional roots of disease and how to truly get to these roots with patients. When I've tried to get to a patient's root emotions and beliefs underlying their illness/life I've often felt I was not able to facilitate or help bring them to such an awareness. Dr. Moshe's course provides you with a very clear framework to work from, and although – as he portrays – it is an art to counsel this way, the way he teaches it makes it feel doable and not overwhelming. You will leave the course feeling ready to start using these tools immediately! Can't say enough good things!

Dr. Willow Langille, ND

For more testimonials about Holistic Counseling – the Course, please visit:

http://www.holistic-counseling.ca/testimonials-holistic-counseling.html

Holistic Counseling

Introducing "The Vis Dialogue"

Breakthrough Healing Method Uniting
The Worlds of Mind-Body Medicine
& Psychology

Holistic Counseling

Introducing "The Vis Dialogue"

Breakthrough Healing Method Uniting
The Worlds of Mind-Body Medicine
& Psychology

Dr. Moshe Daniel Block, ND

**PSYCHE
BOOKS**

Winchester, UK
Washington, USA

First published by Psyche Books, 2016
Psyche Books is an imprint of John Hunt Publishing Ltd., Laurel House, Station Approach,
Alresford, Hants, SO24 9JH, UK
office1@jhpbooks.net
www.johnhuntpublishing.com
www.psyche-books.com

For distributor details and how to order please visit the 'Ordering' section on our website.

Text copyright: Moshe Daniel Block 2015

ISBN: 978 1 78535 209 6
Library of Congress Control Number: 2015949722

A CIP catalogue record for this book is available from the British Library.

Design: Stuart Davies

Printed and bound by CPI Group (UK) Ltd, Croydon, CR0 4YY, UK

We operate a distinctive and ethical publishing philosophy in all
areas of our business, from our global network of authors to
production and worldwide distribution.

CONTENTS

Foreword

"Every drugless practitioner needs a working knowledge of Mental Science," said Benedict Lust, the founder of naturopathic medicine. "The vital organs and functions of the body depend on the nerves for healthy action; the nerves are controlled by the brain, glands, solar plexus and subconscious mind; all of which are made strong or weak, healthy or sickly, normal or abnormal, by the character of our thoughts, emotions and expectations."

Naturopathic texts of the past traditionally placed a lot of focus and emphasis on the psychological, mental, emotional, and spiritual states of the patient and found these to be crucial in the healing process. The practitioner was instructed to apply "mental therapeutics" and "psychological exercises," to energize and balance the body, address the fundamental cause of disease, and to help repair and restore the healthy functioning of the vital force. The modern version of this approach is the clinical field of mind-body medicine and the cutting-edge work of Dr. Moshe Daniel Block ND, contained in *Holistic Counseling – Introducing "The Vis Dialogue."*

Current clinical and scientific research in the field of epigenetics, psycho-neuro immunology and neuroplasticity validates the importance of the mind-body connection that our naturopathic ancestors guided us towards. Dr. Moshe's approach and teachings contained in *Holistic Counseling* represent a much-needed "mental therapeutics" and "psychological exercises" of a naturopathic text for the present and future. The book both remains true to long expressed core traditional naturopathic principles and philosophy and at the same time presents practically applied and integrated powerful and effective healing therapeutics. With this book, Dr. Moshe would make our founders proud and will make all naturopathic physicians, other health-care practitioners and their patients filled with gratitude as they use his guidance to support getting well, healing, and curing.

Dr. Moshe is a philosopher, a "wounded" healer, a psychologist, a scientist, a teacher, a guide, a therapist, a shaman, a compassionate and wise spiritual being all rolled into one. He is a pioneering, true naturopathic physician, honoring and following in the footsteps of his ancestors and beyond, even expanding the essential teachings. His understandings and insights parallel my own 30-year plus career specializing in mind-body integrative medicine. And as a kindred spirit and co-pioneer, I can empathize with and appreciate what Dr. Moshe had to go through to stay true to the essence of his teachings amidst a profession that was struggling with its identity within an evolving and changing health care landscape. We first came to learn of each other as our articles were published in the same mind-body medicine issue of NDNR, a Naturopathic Journal. I was very happy and excited to find a kindred spirit and mind-body medicine and psychology oriented naturopathic colleague. Interestingly, his use of questions at the heart of his approach was interestingly similar to my own, like a parallel universe, as over time I too would discover and utilize asking living questions as a key component and at the heart of my work with clients.

In combining mind-body medicine and psychology in a nature cure naturopathic medicine context, *Holistic Counseling* offers much needed practical tools and perspectives for physicians and patients alike, bringing the roots of natural healing to life. In the spirit of Benedict Lust, he provides, "a working knowledge of mental science" in the search for finding and treating the underlying cause and activating the vital force. His therapeutic approach embodies the words of Norman Vincent Peale, "Every problem has in it the seeds of its own solution. If you don't have any problems, you don't get any seeds." For Dr. Moshe, pain and illness is the teacher that contains the seeds providing the opportunity to find meaning and healing.

"Holistic Counseling is a method of counseling that involves simple but most powerful principles. The main idea or principle of Holistic Counseling is that, by asking questions in a non-directive fashion, we help a person see the answers to their own problems, as those answers lie within themselves. It is a method which helps a person see the innermost workings of their mind, and how their false ideas are trapping them, impacting their body, and making them sick." Dr. Moshe

His emphasis is on the consciousness of the patient, their attitudes, beliefs, emotions and thoughts in relation to their disease and as a key element in their path leading to healing. He works with where the healing can be found, looking deep within, where the real self is brought forth from the person's own mind and heart. The mind-body medicine that Dr. Moshe teaches emphasizes the important role of the physician to guide the journey, but only in *supporting* the conscious awareness, choice and active engagement in the self-healing process of the patient. His work and words are authentic and speak from deep inner truth, wisdom and compassion, emanating from and gained and realized in his own evolutionary transformational journey facing and healing from a chronic disease, myasthenia gravis.

He embodies the "wounded healer," Carl Jung speaks about. "The doctor is effective only when he himself is affected." The lessons learned and earned in that health challenge is the experience that spurred him forward to share his hard-fought wisdom of healing himself with others. And now offering this wonderful, wise, and important work to a larger audience of practitioners and patients alike, this book is for anyone seeking authentic healing, wholeness and freedom from suffering.

All healing is self-healing – the journey home to your true self. *Holistic Counseling* provides a roadmap and a how-to manual for this journey, instructions and skillful means in mind-body medicine and psychology applied holistically.

As Larry Dossey MD has said, "Healing is not a matter of

setting the molecules straight, it is a matter of helping the one in need of healing into an experience of wholeness." Those who work with Dr. Moshe, and/or read this book and apply his teachings will have precisely that sort of an experience of wholeness.

Dr. Moshe speaks of healing with *awareness itself* as the agent of healing. As a homeopathic oriented naturopath, Dr. Moshe practices homeopathy and has seen cures occur even without a remedy, allowing the awareness, wisdom and acceptance of painful truth to be the healer. From Indian philosopher Krishnamurti, "It is the truth which liberates, not your effort to be free".

"I have seen cases cured of serious physical illness, like my own and many others with myasthenia gravis and other conditions, by awareness alone, without administering a single remedy. I have helped many people be drug free and symptom free simply by first helping them discover their underlying core belief that led to their illness, and then helping them make a new choice about who they are and how they want to be. So Holistic Counseling can be applied to just about any form of illness." Dr. Moshe

For real and transformative healing, bringing to life the deeper wisdom of naturopathic philosophy, Dr. Moshe's words are a beacon of light and provide an often-missing essential ingredient in the growing movement of holism, integrative medicine, functional medicine, natural therapies, mind-body medicine, lifestyle and wellness. In *Holistic Counseling*, Dr. Moshe ensures this important dimension and ingredient of care is fully addressed and integrated, focusing on the underlying cause and activating the Vis (The Healing Power of Nature).

"This book is full of information and philosophy necessary to prepare oneself for the obstacles, difficulties, and opposition one faces while applying the principles of real holistic medicine." Dr. Moshe

Dr. Paul Epstein, Naturopathic physician
Mind-body Medicine Pioneer
Author of *Happiness Through Meditation*
Co-founder Isreal Center for Mind-Body Medicine
www.DrPaulEpstein.com

Acknowledgments

I'd like to thank all of my patients who have had the courage to follow a path much less traveled and who have taught me so much through our successes and failures together. Without you, none of this would be possible.

To all of the students that have taken Holistic Counseling – The Course, thank you for your beautiful attention and feedback that have helped this work spread and grow.

I'd like to thank Barry Neil Kaufman for teaching me the Optiva Dialogue at the Option Institute in Massachusetts in 1995, which became the foundation for developing and broadening the Vis Dialogue.

To all of the teachers who have been true to Holism and Vitalism through my studies, in and out of the classroom, through the years, your courage and wisdom are gifts beyond measure. Without you, none of this could be possible.

I'd like to thank my parents, John and Trish Block, who supported me through my Naturopathic medical studies, and helped guide me to return to my studies during the three times I tried to quit the program.

I'd like to thank my wife, Svea, who recognized the value of the process of questions I used in practice even when I didn't and who was the original inspiration that encouraged me to begin teaching Holistic Counseling before it was even conceived as a course. I want to thank her also for going over this book with me and helping to edit.

I'd also like to thank the Creator, the Great Orchestrator of this world and the Healing Power of Nature, for this profound, mysterious, challenging, and magnificent life, without whom *none* of this could be possible.

Introduction to Holistic Counseling

The medicine of today is mostly based on a model that seeks to treat the symptoms of disease at the level of the body, and not the whole person, nor at the root cause. Called the allopathic model of medicine, this form of treatment is dominant in conventional medicine. What has been rather startling for me to recognize through my years of study and practice is how prevalent this model of medicine also is in the alternative medicine world. The philosophical principles of Naturopathic medicine point to a much more holistic model of medicine. These principles are written on the walls of the colleges, and on the websites of practitioners, yet are taught very little, understood less, and barely applied in practice. The allopathic model comprises the principle that the knowledge for healing, as well as the application of the treatment, must come from the doctor, and is therefore outside of the patient. This method leaves the patient in the dark about what has led to their problem and is one of the greatest factors that cripple the ability of those who endeavor to heal their patients via way of the allopathic model. The same is true for most forms of counseling and psychology. The idea that the knowledge of what will help the patient comes via the authority of the counselor or psychologist through advice and the application of different suggested exercises and life changes. The increasing quantity and severity of the illness of the world is truly crying out for medicine much more aligned with Nature. People are dying, literally, to understand themselves better. What most do not know, patients and practitioners alike, is that the most lasting and powerful way to heal a patient's pathology, whether it be mental, emotional, and/or physical, is by helping them have an epiphany to recognize the root cause of their problem. People are dying for the true philosophical principles of holistic medicine to be carried forward into practice. Holistic

Counseling is a form of counseling based on philosophical principles of holism that is the answer to the dilemma that the world faces in its ineffective forms of medicine.

Holistic Counseling is a method of counseling that involves simple but most powerful principles.

The main idea or principle of Holistic Counseling is that, by asking questions in a non-directional fashion, we help a person see the answers to their own problems, as those answers lie within themselves. It is a method which helps a person see the innermost workings of their mind, and how their false ideas are trapping them, impacting their body, and making them sick. Holistic Counseling is also about holism in general, and both the course and this book are designed to discuss and explore holism so that it can be embraced and utilized in practice.

If there ever was a time that needed true holistic medicine, it is now.

The world is so very advanced in its illness and people need so much healing – they are so disconnected from themselves and filled with horrible toxic energies. You can intervene in a person's life and ask them questions to get them to see the mistakes that are making their lives a living hell. Even in one session it is possible to arrive at an awareness with a person that truly changes their life. Those who practice Holistic Counseling are told by their patients that one session alone is like having many years of different forms of counseling and psychotherapy. The depths that can be arrived at in a Holistic Counseling session are truly remarkable.

I began developing Holistic Counseling in 2000, when I first started seeing patients. I based Holistic Counseling on a technique called *The Optiva Dialogue* that I had learned from Barry Neil Kaufman at the Option Institute in Massachusetts. It was in 1995 when *The Optiva Dialogue* helped me have a major breakthrough in my own health. It was the first year that I was diagnosed with myasthenia gravis, a rare, allegedly potentially fatal, incurable, and progressive auto-immune disease. I had quite pronounced paralysis of my tricep muscles, diplopia (double vision), and weakness in other muscle groups. *The Optiva Dialogue*, much like Holistic Counseling, is based on asking non-directional and non-judgmental questions. It was all that I needed. The practitioner that worked with me asked me a series of questions that helped me go deeper and deeper into my subconscious mind, until we arrived at a major part of the root of my illness. Like the opening at the bottom of a funnel, the questions circled around and finally converged on the special question, what I call, *the right question*, which helped unlock the biggest problem I was carrying. I had answered one of the questions of the dialoguer – "Because I need to be perfect." And then their next question did the trick. "What makes you feel you need to be perfect?" That was it. That caused my whole world to spin. This basic premise, held onto so potently in my mind, had never been questioned, and remained unchallenged, laying as the foundation for so much stress and inner turmoil. Believing that I needed to be perfect, I would judge myself harshly against the backdrop of perfection when I thought I had erred or done something that I deemed unworthy of the mark of perfection. As self-imposed and insubstantial as it was, it nevertheless controlled my life and had led to my illness. I knew this without a doubt after I was asked the question, "What makes you think you need to be perfect?" because I decided, at that moment, that it was not such a good idea, it was not a necessary reality, and by that simple focus, I was able to release the belief. With that came a spontaneous healing. Life force flowed into my body. My eyes cleared up and my arms swelled with blood and strength. It was a moment I will never forget.

It was such a gift to be asked "the right question." There are many good questions we can ask people to get them to recognize where their beliefs are limiting their reality, and then there is the question that is poised at the threshold of discovery and does the trick to open up a larger and healthier world than the one the person had formed around their minds that limited them and made them sick.

Not everyone will have spontaneous healing when made aware of the beliefs that are making them suffer. But both Holistic Counseling – The Course, and this book are designed to offer awareness and exercises for how to deal with many manners of stuckness of mind, emotion, and body, to help a person evolve in their lives toward freedom and health.

I have written this book to complement Holistic Counseling – The Course, not to strictly act as a stand-alone teaching tool to enable someone to be able to carry out the process of Holistic Counseling, without the course. I have also written this book to ensure that I can convey as much of the knowledge I have gained through my experiences as possible. Even though I attempt to share as much as I can during each weekend course, each class is different and the knowledge that emerges is not always the same as others. Also, time is limited, and it becomes impossible to deal with all the vital topics that arise in this area. Through these pages, you will see as much as I can possibly share on the topic. Having said that, some information that is witnessed during the course, cannot be conveyed through these pages. Watching live cases and practicing the dialogue are essential to grasping the Vis Dialogue. Also, certain information, due to its subtle nature, is much better shared live, in person, than via a book.

Receiving Holistic Counseling is most definitely a gift. It is also a gift to practice, because then we see how much we ourselves are blocked from practicing holistically. Practicing allopathically, i.e. giving 'things' (drugs, supplements, or herbs, etc.) for disease, does not require one's entire being to be present during practice. It is not necessary to be open emotionally when all you have to do is administer 'this' supplement for 'that' condition. But when practicing holistic medicine, and in particular, Holistic Counseling, the practitioner must be open, in mind and heart, or else the patient will not feel comfortable and supported in sharing their innermost painful wounds and misperceptions. And from time to time, more or less frequently, a case will show up where we have a hard time remaining non-directional, or where we simply cannot see what question to ask next to help unlock a person's lock and chain. It is at this time that the practitioner has to look within themselves and ask the question, "What blocked me from helping this person?" Often, it is some wound that the patient carried that triggered a similar wound of the practitioner. And so through difficulty in practice, we as practitioners continue to have our issues revealed to us. This promotes continual growth, "continuing education" in the deepest sense, and it always keeps one humble.

Being a Naturopathic doctor specializing in Homeopathy has really enabled me to evolve *The Optiva Dialogue* and adapt it to working with cases of serious pathology/disease in the body as well as the mental-emotional sphere. People usually associate counseling with sorting out emotional issues, relationship troubles, fear, anxiety, and other non-corporeal issues. But I have seen cases cured of serious physical illness, like my own and many others with myasthenia gravis and other conditions, by awareness alone, without administering a single remedy. I have helped many people be drug free and symptom free simply by first helping them discover their underlying core belief that led to their illness, and then helping them make a new choice about who they are and how they want to be. So Holistic Counseling can be applied to just about any form of illness.

This book is full of information and philosophy necessary to prepare oneself for the obstacles, difficulties, and opposition one faces while applying the principles of real holistic medicine.

Being a Naturopathic doctor *and* homeopath who was sick and had a spontaneous healing experience, has helped me see how the body reflects the mind. When the underlying and also, untrue, belief system is released by no longer choosing to hold it as reality, the body recovers. I use the expression that the body is a faithful puppy dog to the mind. When the mind says "Sit!" the body sits. When the mind chooses, "I am uptight. I have all these emotions bottled up inside me," the body responds by creating high blood pressure. When the mind says, "I have to hold on to all of this crap," the body reflects that via manifesting constipation. It is a one-to-one relationship and often, after the physical symptoms of the disease are explored in depth, as we do in Holistic Counseling, there can be seen such an accurate reflection between the physical symptoms and the belief systems that led to those symptoms. It is truly remarkable. In my case I had a very clear understanding shown about auto-immune disease. In such an illness, the immune system is literally turned against itself. We thus always find in auto-immune illness, with perhaps a very few exceptions, that the person, in some way, is attacking themselves. For me, I did so because it was my way of punishing myself for not being perfect. "You idiot!" I would say to myself. The intention there was that I was bad. Thinking I was bad, I attacked myself mentally and emotionally. The faithful puppy dog in my body responded in kind and my immune system turned towards my neuro-muscular junction. (The exact part of the body the immune system would attack in an auto-immune disease is an interesting topic and worthy of discussion and investigation.) When the source of attacking myself, i.e. needing to be perfect, was released, my body released the need to emulate the mind and I was healed. There was nothing wrong with my muscles, nor my immune system. There was certainly nothing wrong with my thymus gland. When one understands holism and how effectively healing it is, the thought of cutting out the thymus gland (thymectomy) in cases of myasthenia gravis, which is still largely practiced today in the conventional medical approach, is so completely barbaric and erroneous, it is really no different from the now obsolete medical interventions like bloodletting in cases of fever, seizure, lung infections and other reasons, or drilling

12

holes in peoples' heads to let out the demons in cases of severe headache. There is also nothing wrong with the colon in constipation. No need to treat it directly as if it were defective. The more one practices holistically, and sees the body respond directly to changes in the mental-emotional sphere, it becomes quite obvious how very little those who practice strictly allopathically understand about the workings of The Healing Power of Nature. In time, as holism becomes more and more adopted by our world, many of the practices of modern medicine will be considered barbaric, much in the way that we now consider drilling holes in a person's head for headaches to be a rather misguided form of medicine.

This is a glimpse into true holism, where the mind and body are one, and the body responds to the mis-thought of the mind by emulating it in its own realm. And this is another great gift we can bring people, to help them make a connection between how their body got sick and what has been going on in their conscious, but mostly subconscious, mind.

Determining what is true and untrue in a case, and in reality in general, is a sensitive and often-times touchy subject, due to some of the organized religions that have attempted to force ideas of God and Creation on people, dictating what is true and what is not. I will not be forcing any beliefs onto anyone, yet my own experiences and practice have shown me that there is an importance in recognizing a Universal Truth that permeates all of creation and when we align our thoughts with it, there is health and harmony. We can say we are living in harmony with The Healing Power of Nature. This is synonymous with The Great Spirit, the Creator, and God. I will address this topic in greater depth in this book.

The Healing Power of Nature is a mystery. A great divine mystery. There are medicines that emanate from that mystery. These are subtle medicines that one can continue to study one's entire life. As one practices them, the basic principles they learned in their introductory lessons about these subtle medicines do not change. They deepen. They grow deeper roots and the branches of understanding reach out to be able to catch more light of wisdom. On such a path, one must tune into this mysterious Healing Power of Nature, and by walking such a path, the practitioner is healed.

The physician is only a servant of Nature, not her master. Therefore, it behooves medicine to follow the will of Nature. Paracelsus

Then there are medicines which are not based on principles of Holism and working in harmony with Nature, but rather, based on control, where the doctor plays God, where the practitioner finds all the solutions for the patient and is falsely responsible for the patient's health. This sort of medicine practiced in control is in total contrast to working with The Healing Power of Nature. Holistic Counseling is a medicine that works in harmony with The Healing Power of Nature. It, as other subtle medicines, like homeopathy, has such very simple principles. They are the easiest to grasp initially, "Like cures like" for homeopathy, and "Ask simple, non-directional questions to get to the root cause of disease" for Holistic Counseling, but are the hardest to practice at first. To practice effectively requires experience, much reflection, a dedication to The Healing Power of Nature, and a willingness to let go of the need to be the one who knows what is right for a patient, the one who is in control.

Practicing Holistic Counseling is not easy. Most beginners of Holistic Counseling find it very difficult to be non-directional in asking questions. Everyone makes this mistake at first. As a practitioner begins to ask questions, it may seem to the practitioner that they know what the patient has to see to be liberated from their issues and illness. So they begin directing the patient by asking leading questions to "help them see" what they are missing. In other words, the question itself contains the "answer" the patient is looking for. This form of counseling is not nearly as effective as the way in which we ask non-directional questions in Holistic Counseling. Being non-directional requires a form of discipline and importantly, a trust in the process and a trust in the patient, believing that they can find their own answers, and that when they do so, it will be that much more rewarding and healing in the long run than just essentially telling them what their problem is. We are quite indoctrinated into the belief that the doctor is responsible for helping the patient and the doctor knows best. This dynamic is unfortunately at play in most healing settings and both patient and doctor can easily fall into the role of "fix me doctor" for the patient, and "I am like God in knowing what is right for you" for the doctor. In Holistic Counseling, it is much more harmonious with The Healing Power of Nature when we simply provide the right setting for our patients to be their own healers. This requires the practitioner to release their own ego and their own need to rescue the patient, which is another way in which practicing holistically is very healing for practitioner as well as the patient.

All in all, practicing Holistic Counseling is a most wonderful endeavor. Each case has such a beautiful tapestry of struggles and themes that have permeated the person's life. These patterns or "threads" that a belief system has entwined in a person's life are fascinating. It seems to be that each one could have a book written about it. To help reveal that scheme to the patient is a true privilege and honor. To then witness the positive healing effects it has in their life is rewarding beyond words.

Part I – Philosophical Background to Holistic Counseling

The Six Main Principles of the Philosophy of Naturopathic and Holistic Medicine and Introducing, the Seventh

1 First of all, to do no harm.
2 To heal the whole person
3 To act in cooperation with The Healing Power of Nature.
4 To address the fundamental cause of disease.
5 To heal each person as an individual
6 Doctor as teacher

When these six points of the philosophy of Naturopathic medicine are explored, it becomes very clear that Naturopathic medicine is based entirely on well thought out principles of Holism.

7 Physician, Heal Thyself! – A vitally important principle of Holism that we will explore through the book.

Let's take a look at each of the Principles of the Philosophy.

Chapter 1

First of All, Do No Harm.

This is a principle shared with conventional medicine. Its meaning is obvious, yet the potential to do harm is at times, subtle and not as obvious as if we, for instance, give a supplement or herbal formula that has ingredients that are contraindicated for a certain condition and cause direct damage from it. We must know when we are in over our heads in a given case and need to refer, and when we need to send a patient to the Emergency room. When we work to treat the symptoms of disease and not the root cause, there is a worsening of the disease at the level of the Vital Force, and this is a form of harm. When we practice counseling allopathically, we offer a lot of advice, we tell the patient what they wish to hear. We can also cause harm by the dependence we create in the patient, and also the advice we thought was accurate but was misleading. When we work holistically and in harmony with Nature, we tend to do no harm, so fear around this topic is unnecessary, but mindfulness and awareness is always important.

Chapter 2

To Heal the Whole Person

The Four Levels of the Whole Person

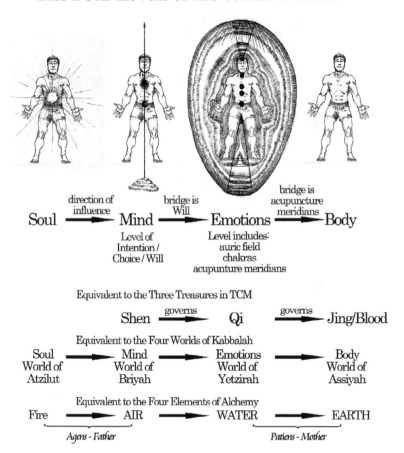

Soul →(direction of influence)→ Mind →(bridge is Will)→ Emotions →(bridge is acupuncture meridians)→ Body

Mind: Level of Intention / Choice / Will

Emotions: Level includes: auric field, chakras, acupuncture meridians

Equivalent to the Three Treasures in TCM

Shen →(governs)→ Qi →(governs)→ Jing/Blood

Equivalent to the Four Worlds of Kabbalah

Soul World of Atzilut → Mind World of Briyah → Emotions World of Yetzirah → Body World of Assiyah

Equivalent to the Four Elements of Alchemy

Fire → AIR → WATER → EARTH

Agens - Father   *Patiens - Mother*

Picture 1 – The Four Levels of the Whole Person

In Picture 1, I depict four-dimensional "worlds" or realities that are equivalent to the four dimensions of the "whole person" widely accepted in Naturopathic medicine. I have depicted some additional similarities spanning other traditions to demonstrate the universality or similarities found in this topic. The understanding of the four dimensions of the human being, along with direction of influence is very important in understanding Holism.

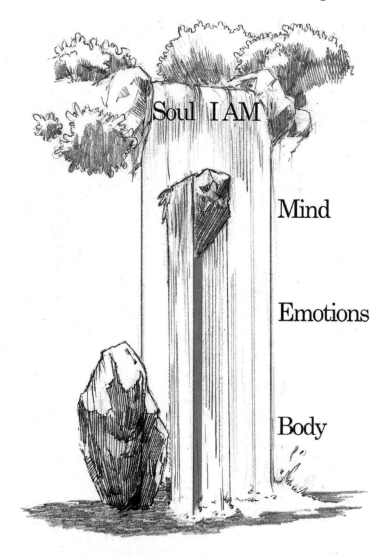

Picture 2 – The Direction of Influence of the four Dimensions of the Whole Person

It is at the soul level where we derive our origins. It is at soul level where our "I AM" statement is pronounced. At the soul level, we sit in a world of infinite healing energy, where The Healing Power of Nature is at its most pure and highest vibrational frequency.

From the soul emanates all life, all vitality. All energies of Nature trickle down to the other three-dimensional worlds that are slower and lower in vibration. One can call them "more dense."

In Picture 2, the waterfall represents the energies that work their way down to the three lower worlds, originating from the world of soul. On the right-hand side of the picture, when there is nothing that interferes with the I AM statement of a soul, the mind is supplied with free-flowing uninhibited and healthy energy from the Universe, from the source of all life, the Creator. We say that in such a state all things are in harmony. The emotions and body will happily reflect the nature of the soul and the mind, all in ways that resonate with and mirror the soul's I AM state.

The Mind and False Belief Systems – The Fundamental Cause of Disease

"Only the mind is capable of error. The body can act wrongly only when it is responding to mis-thought."[1]

On the left-hand side of Picture 2, we see that a rock, at the level of the mind, is impeding the flow of the vital life force that emanates from the soul. As a result, the emotional world and the physical world (body) will equally be blocked from the supply of the vital life force. This is how disease begins in a person. First the mind adopts some form of false idea (called a negative belief system) that is not in harmony with the I AM statement of the soul. This gets in the way or impedes the natural flow of emanation from the higher world to the lowest. In simple terms, health comes from being oneself. Disease results in believing something about the self which is incorrect and then living by that false belief.

It is because the belief system that a person chooses to believe is false that it impedes the flow of life force. A belief or way of thinking that is in harmony with the state of I AM at the soul level, will simply work in harmony, flow, and be a part of the source of Truth from the soul. One can say such a belief in the mind that is in harmony is not even an active or willful state of mind, but rather that it emanates from the soul and is effortless. It is therefore, take note, not even a choice. It is more like a reflection of the soul, and a way of the mind "knowing" one's I AM statement. That is an effortless form of observation of what is. Here we see that we did not create ourselves and life is therefore more about discovery of self and then *allowing ourselves to be who we really are*.

One way we discover who we are is by recognizing what we are not. We know what we are not by choosing to believe something false about ourselves and discovering that it really doesn't work for us. It doesn't work because when we believe something false about who we are and about Nature Itself, we become sick in mind, emotions and body. This is where choice, i.e. free will, comes into the picture.

Choice, i.e. free will, comes into the picture when a person chooses to adopt and hold a false set of ideas and beliefs in their mind. It is important to note that within the healing process, the person must make a willful choice to unchoose these false beliefs. A simpler way of saying this is that in order to heal, a person must let go of these false beliefs. Such is a choice to unchoose or release a false thought. It is like having a fist closed around the false thought in the mind and all it takes in healing is to open up the hand and let drop what has been held. In disease, we must hold onto it in this way with the will of the mind because it is not a natural occurrence in the mind. What is natural does not need to be held onto in such a fashion. What is natural emanates from

Nature. This is true Nature. That is why a very healthy person aligned with their I AM statement and truly being themselves, is not very "stuck up in their mind." True Nature is Truth and needs only to be observed emanating from the soul. Truth emanates from the Creator and so we can say that at the soul level, we are One with the Creator; only that which is false and that which causes disease needs to be held on to with the will of the mind. It is as simple as that, though, as we will explore further in this book, not always easy. All true healing is simple. This does not make it easy.

What we also observe in recognizing this cascade and direction of influence, is that the emotions and the body take on the form of the belief system because each of the lower worlds, emotions and body, are reflections of the higher world of the mind (and the mind, in one's true state, is the reflection of the higher world of soul). What we observe in Holistic Counseling, which confirms this reflection between the mind, emotions, and body, is that people will describe their illness in the very same terms and with the same analogies as the false choices that led to the disease. The reason for that is the mind and emotions are centered in the body, which has all emanated from the soul. There are not really four worlds but rather one continuum of life force that has different states of density. So when a person describes how they feel about their illness and what it makes them do, or not do, it is naturally a reflection of the mental-emotional unhealthy patterns that led to the disease in the body. There is no separation there. Only the illusion of separation. And for the purpose of describing these subtle relationships and directions of influence, we speak about the continuum in four stages or worlds.

We see in Traditional Chinese Medicine (TCM) that *"The Three Treasures"* also demonstrate this direction of influence (see Picture 1). The Shen (Mind) governs the Qi (which is on the same dimensional level as the world of emotions) which governs the

Blood (which is the same world as the physical body). A problem at the level of Shen will reflect a problem in the flow of Qi which will influence the flow of blood. For a change to occur to the body there must be a problem in the flow of Qi. For there to be a problem with the Qi, there must be an issue with the Shen (mind) for this is the direction of influence. The wise observer of Nature optimizes The Healing Power of Nature by working in harmony with this direction of influence. So the most effective and lasting way of healing in chronic illness is to address the problem where it lies at its deepest level – that is at its fundamental cause, which is in the world of the mind, and in particular, involves releasing those false belief systems that block the flow of the natural emanation of life force. Trying to heal the body in chronic illness by addressing the symptoms at the level of the body represents a gross misunderstanding of the direction of influence of Nature. Trying to address the cause of chronic illness at the level of the body could be likened to standing at the base of the waterfall and trying to push up at the water in an attempt to prevent the problem at the lowest level.

"All material means that you accept as remedies for bodily ills are restatements of magic principles."[2]

"Since the body is only an effect of thoughts in the mind, any "problems" in the body must also be an effect of thought. If we try to fix the body at the level of form, which is the level of effect, we are trying to heal the body using inappropriate means. This is called magic, which is trying to make illusions seem real. They are attempts to make the illusions of the ego seem real by trying to fix its 'problems' with something in the physical world instead of healing the thoughts in the mind which is the real cause of every problem."[3]

Emotions – The Watery Medium

The method of Holistic Counseling is largely applied through the mind because we are endeavoring to remove the fundamental cause in the waterfall flow of the Vital Force which are the false beliefs we hold in our minds, believing them to be true. So where do the emotions fit into the picture and what is their importance? Surely, there's no doubt that the majority of the patients I work with end up crying during some, and if not, most of our sessions together. And emotions like anger, frustration, guilt, are often more than present in a case. But is crying necessary? Does a patient need to emote in order to effect change in their health, or can the whole dialogue strictly be conducted on the intellectual level and evade the emotional realm?

I have found that in the cases where a patient has contacted the underlying emotion that is associated with and secondary to the inherent beliefs in the subconscious mind, the healing goes much better, faster, and lasts longer. Whether this happens during the appointment, or after while the patient reflects on all they have undergone, or even during their dreams in their sleep, if the stuck energies do not move through the emotional realm, the body will respond much slower.

Health is linked to emotional responsiveness in the face of changing life circumstances and social interactions. The word "e-motion" tells it all – we want to keep our feelings and energy in motion, rather than locking them in our tissues. Sat Dharam Kaur, ND

Why does this happen?

A way of answering this question lies in the art and science of alchemy. Alchemy is an in-depth study of Nature through a most fascinating lens. Some of our ancestors, who were the forebears of Naturopathic medicine and science, like Paracelsus, Sir Isaac Newton, Carl Jung and Robert Boyle, regarded the world through alchemical principles. One of the main focuses of alchemy is the four elements, namely, Fire, Air, Water, and Earth. In some ways, this is literal, and from other perspectives, a lover of Nature learns to discern all the different ways of understanding what an element is and in what form it may appear to us. As I depicted in Picture 1, I have found these four elements to correspond very well to the four dimensions of the human being, namely soul (Fire), mind (Air), emotions (Water), and body (Earth). It is not hard to understand these associations, as the body has a dense nature, like the element of earth. The emotions often feel quite watery, and move in waves, and have often been associated with the water element in Kabbalah, New Age and other forms of writing. The mind has a subtler and invisible quality to it, and can be likened to air. The soul has often been depicted in poetry, in religious literature, and in other ways as fiery.

Alchemy teaches the following tenet which is very important for our present discussion of the importance of the emotions in healing:

Non transire posse ab uno extreme ad alterus ad abseque medio.[4]
Translation from the Latin: One cannot pass from one extreme (thing) to another without an intermediary.

In the book, *The Golden Chain of Homer,* a most definitive text on alchemy, and by many considered the most important book of alchemy, the author Homer, emphasizes this point often. He writes:

For Heaven (Fire) can never become Earth without the inter-mediary of Air and Water, and Earth can never become Heaven without Water and Air as intermediaries between Heaven and Earth. Likewise, Heaven can hardly become Water without Air, and neither can Earth become Air without the agency of the Water.

Heaven is subtle, pure, clear, thin, and volatile; Earth, on the contrary, is coarse, thick, dark, and highly fixed. These two are opposed to each other in consequence of their properties.

26

For if someone wished to unite and coagulate Heaven, the most volatile, with Earth, the most fixed, he could never do it: For the most volatile flies back into its chaos when a little warmth is applied, and it leaves the fixed behind. This occurs in all things thru the whole of nature: The most volatile and the most fixed can never be joined or united without an intermediary.[5]

And here we have our answer about the importance of the emotional realm, because the mind, like Air, is very subtle and, in alchemical terms, quite volatile. We can call it "high in frequency of vibration." The body, like Earth, on the other hand, is much denser and more fixed. The mind cannot affect the body without the medium of the emotions, which is the element of Water. If any chronic disease has become manifest in the body, the emotional world must therefore also equally have become affected and out of balance. So when we are dealing with disease that has become manifest in the body, if we are to see the body heal in the most expedient fashion, once the belief system that is at the root of the disease is released, the emotions must be made to move and also released to bring about full effect of healing.

In alchemy, we can also see the direction of influence. The higher or more volatile elements of Fire and Air are grouped together and considered *Agens* in Latin, which means, the active part. These are considered as Father, or male, or Yang, in the context of the Yin-Yang balance of Nature. Water and Earth, on the other hand, are considered *Patiens,* the passive part. These are considered as the Mother, or female, or Yin.

And herein lies the divide between the male and female. Where the mind lives in the air element, the beliefs that are adopted and held to be true are the active part that translates down through the world of Water and subsequently into the realm of Earth. Both the Water and the Earth are passively influenced by the activity of the mind. What this also means is that we really cannot try to make ourselves feel a certain way about something. Yes, we can suppress our feelings, ignore them and pretend we're not feeling something by using the will of our mind to do so. But we cannot, for instance, make ourselves fall in love with someone that we do not naturally feel attracted to or interested in, and we cannot make ourselves feel happy about a situation that we do not naturally enjoy. Our emotions respond passively in alignment with who we really are, which is our I AM statement, as it emerges from the soul (Fire). If our I AM is a certain way, our emotions respond passively in reflection to the nature of our soul. This cannot be changed. If it were changed, it would be an abomination outside of the harmony of Nature and very unnatural, like a GMO (genetically modified organism) modification to the connection between our soul and emotional makeup.

The mind has the most immediate and quickest influence on the emotions and once the emotions have become affected, they will in turn have an impact on the body, which is a slower effect, due to its denser, more fixed nature.

It should be noted that when we refer to the realm/world of emotions, this is not only describing actual feelings, like joy, sadness, anger, self-esteem, etc. but also that it refers to that level in the human being which also holds the acupuncture meridians, levels of the auric field, and the chakra system (Picture 1). The world of Emotion is the same as the Water element in the relative four worlds of the human being. Just as in The Three Treasures, the mind (Shen) governs the Qi which governs the blood (Jing). In our explanation of the importance of the emotions as being the watery medium between the mind and the body, all the aspects of the human being that dwell in the element of Water, must also move to bring about change in the body. So the Qi and chakras and auric field must move to bring about healing when the Shen's issue is corrected in order to bring about healing to the body. Very often, the Qi and auric field will naturally move when an underlying false belief system is removed.

From this perspective of the multi-dimensional makeup of our nature, the mind exists on the level of intention – a quantum level higher than the auric field, meridians, and chakra system. This is also depicted in Picture 1.

The Divide between the Upper and Lower Worlds in the Human Being

Because of the nature of the world as we have lived in duality, there is a divide between the male and the female. I discuss this in greater depth in a following section. Where the male and female live and conjoin in harmony, there is great love and the end of suffering. That is the goal and the ideal and is possible, although difficult, to achieve. And because there is a divide between the male and the female, we see this also as a divide between the mind, as it exists in the male end of the spectrum, and the emotions and body, as they exist in the female end of the spectrum.

People tend to live centered largely in one area or the other, which creates imbalance and health difficulties. Each has its own problem that needs to be understood properly so that a Holistic Counselor can help such a patient to the greatest degree. So, a person that tends to be very intellectual will hover above their emotions and outside their body. They are thus disconnected from their feelings. However, this does not mean that any false belief that they carry will not influence their Qi system and their emotions. It does and it will. Yet they may remain ignorant of that fact and out of touch with the imbalances that the false belief has caused in their emotions. They simply are out of touch. The sign that something is wrong will become apparent only when the affected cascade has reached the body/Earth level through the medium of Water/emotions/Qi. For sure a dialogue with them takes place where they are most comfortable – in the mind. They may find it difficult to answer any questions that are emotional in nature, like, "How does that feel?" but will have no trouble answering questions that are intellectual in nature, such as, "What makes you think that...?"

In such a case, the practitioner must make it clear that the patient needs to reconnect with their emotions and feelings, even if it takes them some time (weeks, months, or years) to do so. The practitioner can even use these metaphors of the direction of influence to explain how the emotions are very important to bring about a healing on the level of the body. I have seen people who began very intellectual and quite out of touch with their feelings, become much more in touch with their feelings within a few months, or up to a year. For such intellectually-Air-dominant people, they may have a lot of Air signs (Gemini, Libra, Aquarius) and strong Air planetary influence in their astrological chart (Mercury, Venus (its air aspect in Libra), Jupiter), or there may just be a "reason" that they have learned to disconnect from their emotions. It is important to address the very fundamental idea that led them to judge the emotions in the first place. This is best done through the Holistic Counseling Dialogue.

For example, a practitioner can ask the following:

"Where did you get the idea to suppress or disconnect from your emotions?"

Often, the answer is a simple one.

"Emotions were never allowed in my family."

Then, explore that with the patient to help them transition out of that idea.

"Do you want to keep living that way?"

In some cases, a person began to disconnect from their emotions due to a specific traumatic event that was too painful for them to continue feeling. In such cases, the Vis Dialogue helps both to arrive at their core belief and is the way to reconnect from the disconnected emotions, because their entire problem revolves around the suppressed emotions. So, the questions through the mind that bring them to the deepest root of their problem will naturally arrive at the spot of blocked emotions. In such a case, having an upheaval of emotion will greatly help move the energies that have been stuck and that have led to their illness.

In some cases, people choose to judge their emotions because a very emotional person "role-modeled" emotions in such a way which was embarrassing, disgusting, or pathetic to them. They chose to "not be that way" and that meant emotional disconnection. This too must be explored and the *Closing Questions* need to be posed regarding whether or not they wish to continue to suppress their vital emotions due to the misuse or poor role-modeling they observed earlier in life.

Emotional disconnect also poses the greater problem of the patient simply being unaware of how they feel. So, the medium through which they experience inner guidance, intuition, a feeling of moral conscience, aversion to things not good for them, reactions to situations that are unhealthy, is turned off. Such a person can then lead a life which is entirely governed by thinking and not by the feedback system that the world of Water/emotions comprises. What this can look like is a person having no feeling of conscience if what they believe they are doing is right even when it is wrong, in that it is actually unaligned with the Great Capitol T Universal Truth.

A person who is very up in the intellect tends to be very willful in their mind. Their will is strong and it is holding onto thoughts which makes it remain lofty and above the "lower" worlds, which the person has judged, for one reason or another that they cannot "sink" down into. What they need to do is to let go of the overly unbalanced willfulness of the mind (too male) and surrender (female) to the emotions, thus allowing themselves to feel more.

On the other hand, some people tend to dwell too much in the emotions and what they require for their healing is the opposite – they need to use the will of their mind to choose a better way of thinking and be more empowered to change what is not serving them. Just as the person who dwells too much in the mind is unaware of their emotions that are nevertheless present, albeit, in a suppressed and disconnected fashion, the person who is too emotional equally possesses a willfulness in their mind, but it may seem distant and disconnected from them. This is problematic in a Holistic Counseling session and in healing in general, because, for change to occur, the active part, the *Agens*, that is, the mind, must choose to make a change. However, the person that is so governed by emotion has chosen to give up their ability to use the will of their mind to align with and think thoughts that are healthier and happier for them. It is like they are stuck in their passivity. They are drowning in the world of Water – emotion. Recall that the emotions are *Patiens* – the passive part.

And since some patients are passively stuck, the very element they need to make change is distant or disconnected from them. In practice, such a person will often say things like "I don't know" when they are asked to answer an intellectual question like **"What makes you think that?"** Somewhere in life, they may have begun to believe they were stupid. One of their parents may have acted superior intellectually to them and/or belittled them into thinking they could not act adequately on the intellectual level. Alternatively, one of their parents may have been quite domineering and insisted that their way was the only way and any attempt at autonomy by the patient was undermined and met with opposition. That could have affected the person to believe that they cannot decide for themselves. Whatever the case may be, sometimes patients do subsist more comfortably in the emotional, Water element than in the mental, Air element. This may also have to do with their dominant planets being in Water signs (Cancer, Scorpio, Pisces) or having many prominent Water planets (Moon, Pluto, Neptune) in their astrological birth chart. Whatever the cause of the ideas or original wounding that led them to choose to be intellectually passive needs to be addressed through the Vis Dialogue just as any other belief system that is unhealthy and harmful to them.

"What made you begin to think you are incapable of deciding for yourself?" and from there the dialogue will unfold.

Some people are naturally more emotional than intellectual and vice versa. That is a normal variation of Nature and to be expected – although the most balanced people will be the most in harmony, and thus, the most happy and healthy.

Our standard education has been largely to blame for some of the problems we face in either extreme that we have discussed here – that is, either too intellectual or too emotional. When a child that tends naturally toward the emotional, creative side of things is forced into a program that is mostly intellectually dominant, and the grades suffer as if it were the very thing that determined if the child was good or bad, it imparts the idea that the child is no good at the intellectual pursuit, and sometimes, in life and society in general. Instead, if the education system, as in some forms of the schooling that do exist, like Waldorf and Montessori schools, encouraged the natural inclinations and gifts of the child, it would result in emotionally, creatively dominant children who could then also learn to harness the power of their intellect more while being encouraged in their natural strengths. It would also promote intellectually dominant children to learn to be more in touch with their feelings, while they are encouraged to do what comes naturally to them in the intellect.

Back from this digression to Holistic Counseling and emotions as the watery medium. It is mostly for those who are intellectually dominant and who have learned to suppress their emotions that need to learn to evoke the emotional realm in order to bring about a healing and change in the body, as one cannot go from one extreme (mind to body) to the other without a medium. The problem of the emotionally dominant person is of a different kind, where they have to be brought to the awareness of what led them to disconnect from their ability to think and to choose according to who they really are. However, since we are such complicated beings, it is possible that one person can actually exhibit both extremes and tendencies. That is, in one aspect of their lives they are intellectually dominant and the emotion is suppressed, and then, in another, they can be stuck in their emotions and unable to "rise above" to use their mind as a vehicle of movement, change, and alignment with their true nature. Such a split could be seen in patients with Borderline Personality Disorder, Bipolar, or in people who exhibit these divided and split tendencies without any diagnosis.

And regardless of which dominance a person leans towards, every person has a mind and emotions. I know that sounds funny because of its obviousness. It is simply to illustrate the fact that the mind is always active in a situation as well as the emotions. The question is therefore, how much of a shroud or disconnect or suppression has been built up surrounding each area? The more of a shroud, the more of a disconnect. Each creates its own dilemma.

There is an advantage regarding the emotional field that can help lead to clues in the mental field. Often, mental beliefs and thought patterns have become so deeply buried in the subconscious that a person is completely out of touch with them. They are unaware of these thoughts, but the emotions still speak louder than words and clearer than the thoughts, since the thoughts are buried and out of conscious awareness. So the emotions will give an insight into what those belief systems are because the emotions are the "congealed" or "denser" watery energetic forms of the mental, Air element beliefs. The Air is a subtler form of an element. It can barely be seen. It is also, for the most part, invisible, except when one can see the powerful effects it has through the wind; whereas water is more tangible, obvious. It can be seen, felt, and touched; air, less so. And so it is with the relationships between the mind's thoughts in Air, and the emotion's feelings in Water. The thoughts congeal into the feelings, and so, even if one is unable to pinpoint an exact thought or belief, by going into the emotions, one begins to stir and evoke the thoughts. As an alchemist stirs up his/her matter with fire and motion, the liquid mediums volatilize into the realm of Air. As feelings are stirred up, they will yield thoughts. *They are like liquid packages of thought.* When they are focused on by being spoken about, felt, remembered, the beliefs that led to them are volatilized and brought into conscious awareness.

Even in emotionally dominant people, and especially for intellectually dominant people, when we get to the root cause, when the mind moves and shifts and the person is willing and wanting to let go, the emotions have to be encouraged to be felt, experienced, and released for optimal healing to take effect.

If the emotion doesn't move, it will make it easier for the person to return to the false belief system and subsequent actions that support it, because they still feel the same, blocked, unhappy, unhealthy way inside. I see this often in practice as do all practitioners who are mindful of these processes in their patients. When asked, **"Do you believe your belief system is the truth?"** often a patient will say, "No, but I feel it is." This is a very case-in-point demonstration of how the mind can operate independently of the emotions. We can also say that due to some chronically held belief system, the emotions passively took on the feeling of the belief. That is, the *Agens* of the mind, influenced the *Patiens* of the emotion, so that the lower, less subtle one was the passive reflection of the more subtle one. It's almost like creating a monster. You've trained a beast to feel a certain way, and now, you instruct it to change and no longer respond in that same way, only, it has become accustomed to your previous instruction and is no longer listening. But don't worry. The beast can be tamed and brought back into useful service to the whole person. And what I recommend is that the person continues to focus mentally on the change in the belief and to perform the corresponding healthy action even though they may feel a strong tug of the emotion back into the disease. This is important. One must make the choice that is aligned with their true nature despite how they may feel inside. With continual focus on the rightful action (more on this in Chapter 22 *Rightful Action for Correction*), the right word, the healing will take place over time until there is no longer any need for determined focus.

Sometimes, when you ask a patient, *"Do you want to keep living this way?"* the whole kit and caboodle moves at the same time. The thought changes, and it pushes the old false belief out, and along with it, the old unhealthy, unhappy feeling that accompanies the false belief goes with it, often with a great gusto of tears, heat, coughing, burping, sighing, and other effects to show that the trapped energies in the emotions have moved out. In such a case, any physical pathology that has manifested as a result of the false belief and reflecting negative emotions, will be able to recover much more quickly than if the mind alone, and without the emotions, changes.

It should be noted that if a person can stay with the change of belief and keep supporting it and nurturing it, that even if the emotions do not readily shift, in time, the person will heal and recover. This is due to the fact that the old, false emotion that was passively supplied by the false belief system no longer has a source to feed it, and it will dry up and eventually disappear. This will then give room for the Qi to move back into the space and heal the body through the medium of Water. This phenomenon is discussed later in the metaphor of the two cabooses. When the source of the fuel that was feeding the disease is removed, the momentum of the caboose of disease slows and eventually stops. The brunt of the difficulty and the risk, however, occurs during the tender and fragile transition time that occurs before the emotion has time to move and where the person still feels the duality between what they are newly choosing to believe and how they feel. It is then that the most slips can occur. A person will go to your office, you will help them change their mind then they return home, still feeling the same. They may allow their mind to keep falling into line with the stuck emotion of the old belief and the false belief system falls back into place and all the negative behavior and life choices that accompany it. It's then that a patient may decide the healing is not working and choose an allopathic solution to remove their symptoms.

It is for this reason that techniques, therapies, and strategies, along with homework, are a very good idea to implement in order to ensure that the medium of Water moves to allow the changes in the mind to reach the body. Once the body shifts, and is healed, it is a sure sign that the world of emotions (which includes emotions themselves as well as the Qi, meridians, and auric field) have equally responded to the release of the false belief. But until then, it is important to encourage the person to contact their feelings, to feel, to cry, to rage, to express frustration, disappointment, how it feels to be neglected, abandoned, suppressed, judged, shunned. When these feelings are acknowledged, they are given space, and thus they move. When they move, the Qi moves and the body can shift as well, just as the waves of the ocean move the sandy beach of the shore. This allows the body to release that which is not healthy for it.

A practitioner can simply sit with the patient and encourage them to feel. Give it space. Don't try to get rid of it, just let it be. When negative emotions are felt in conjunction with the release of false beliefs and the adoption of the good healthy beliefs, they do not stay long. They are re-experienced and then they are gone.

Here is where "Physician, Heal Thyself!" is of utmost importance. How can you guide a patient to accept and feel their painful emotion if you, yourself, have not done so? The energies that fly between people when they are in close communication are tremendous. When that dynamic is in a healing setting, it is all the more powerful and impactful. If the practitioner is sitting in judgment of their own sadness, that, in and of itself, can be blocking the patient from releasing their own sadness that stands between the shift of mind and body. If the practitioner believes anger is bad and should be suppressed or swept under the carpet, how can a patient be expected to accept their own anger in the presence of such a practitioner? I often see practitioners say they are getting stuck in helping their patients contact and resolve their emotions, or they are having difficulty with the intensity and negativity of their patients' emotions, and it always comes back to the fact that the practitioner has issues with their own emotions.

Interestingly, since the Earth element is neighboring the element of Water, by moving the body, one can also inspire a movement in the emotions, especially if a person's focus is to get their emotions moving through exercise. Here the level of fitness reflects how labile the emotional field can be. It is a general principle and not an absolute one, because a person who is out of shape, can easily contact their feelings. However, in the case of someone who has had long-standing stuck emotions, if the Earth shakes, rattles, and rolls, it will help move things along on the emotional front. Being in shape, therefore, is important to move healing along and keep things flowing for both the Earth and Water elements.

Some techniques and activities that are good for moving the emotions are:

- EFT – Emotional Freedom Technique.
- Body Work, Massage, Osteopathy, and other forms of body work.
- Reiki and hands of healing.
- Breathwork.
- Martial Arts (all) but especially Tai Qi and Qi Gong.
- Acupuncture, which can move the Qi, to accompany the change in belief and can even be targeted specifically to the

affected organs of the emotions and beliefs in question. For e.g.: anger, work with liver points, sadness, lungs, etc.
• Trauma-Tension Release Exercises ala David Berceli.
• Exercise where a person focuses on allowing their feelings while they jog, bike, swim, hit a heavy bag, do Yoga, etc.
• The "Hold it For Longer" Technique (ala this author, me)
• Punch a pillow to get the anger out.
• Sing out the emotions. Sing a song that evokes the emotions or make up a song with the words that help to move the emotions.
• Watch a sad, tear-jerker movie to get the sadness out.
• Write a letter to the person who was involved in wounding them. (Send it, or burn it.)
• Journal
• Do Art Therapy

Some of these techniques for getting in touch with one's feelings are carried out through homework that the practitioner gives the patient to do when they go home.

Now onto the next principle of Naturopathic medicine and Holism in general.

Chapter 3

To Act in Cooperation with the Healing Power of Nature

The Healing Power of Nature, that is, *Vis Medicatrix Naturae* (the "Vis" for short), is a great and beautiful mystery that I refer to at various points in this book. I have already begun to share aspects of it in the introduction and the above section of the whole person. Wherever I mention it, I will endeavor to paint a picture of The Vis in such a way that its essence can be understood by the reader, but it will always remain a mystery with which the lover of Nature and healing can continue to develop a deeper relationship.

The Healing Power of Nature is ever present. Like the waves of the oceans washing up on the shore, it is ever at the ready to enter into a person and bring about healing, provided the underlying cause of the illness is addressed and removed. The Healing Power of Nature, like the will of God, does not interfere with free will – that is, with the choices a person is making about the reality of the world we live in. So when we adopt beliefs that are not in harmony with our true nature, they sit as a lump or a block in the flow of life's Vital Force. This blocks out the ever-present, ever-flowing and readily available Healing Power of Nature which is, by its very own essence, in harmony with Nature itself, and, I may add, with The Creator.

So, to choose something untrue to Creation is to set a block in the flow of true nature. This then manifests symptoms in the body that are similar to and that reflect the nature of the belief. For instance, choices of misplaced anger will resonate with those parts of the body "resonant with" anger – that is, the liver, the eyes, certain muscles in the back and the specific chakra related to the domain that the anger is stemming from. Anger at being mistreated which leads to feelings of low self-esteem would affect and block the solar plexus (third) chakra. Anger relating to body image would affect the second chakra and anger related to not being heard would influence the flow of the throat chakra. Sadness affects the lungs, and a person's posture. Fear erodes the energy of the kidneys. These are general principles we know that are derived from our history of observation of the body's response to certain emotions. However, anywhere in the body can store trapped and suppressed emotions as well as be affected by any emotion. It is crucial to allow the body to tell the story of what is affecting the person and not for the practitioner to make assumptions based on the organ, for instance, the liver, and then to state that the a person's liver is sick because they are angry, without that having been revealed naturally through the dialogue.

When we use the Holistic Counseling questions to help establish a connection between a person's illness and the choices they are making, we address the fundamental root cause of the problem. Once it is removed, The Healing Power of Nature aka God/Creator/The Great Spirit, simply comes in to fill in the space previously occupied by the false reality. That is a very simple yet advanced way of working in harmony with The Healing Power of Nature.

Chapter 4

To Address the Fundamental Cause of Disease

It has already been established that the source of chronic illness, that is, the fundamental cause, lies in the false belief systems in the mental world of the Air element. The influence of healing becomes exponentially stronger each higher dimension we travel up. So we can have some effect on the illness in the body by giving physical supplements and drugs (Earth level). But since the cause is not addressed, the symptoms are only suppressed. This actually serves to worsen the Vital Force mistunement (the cause). Inner imbalances and mistunements are actually aided somewhat by being able to have some form of outward expression which takes place in the form of symptoms. And sometimes, we cannot even suppress the symptoms with physical-Earth-element supplements or drugs. The fundamental cause of illness is just too strong and the body does not respond to the selected "material means" that are attempts to correct the problem at the lowest level of its manifestation.

If we move into the world of the Water element, that includes emotions, as well as Qi, chakras, and the auric field, and we attempt to correct the problem in the body, we have a much greater influence, since we have moved a quantum level/dimension higher in the direction of influence of Nature. So, performing acupuncture, Reiki, hands on healing and other modalities that correct illness at the Water level, in the world of emotion, will be much more effective than working strictly at the level of the physical body. However, these modalities still do not address *the fundamental cause*, as in the cause at the deepest point of origin, because that is in the mind. And so they cannot have the deepest and most influential effect on healing.

And here is an important point. There is nothing that can influence the mind to release false belief systems except for a person's conscious choice. This is a general rule that must be understood and respected by the healer and practitioner of Holistic medicine. You can have the best healer do the most wonderful work on a person's energy field, but if that does not somehow influence the patient to let go of the choice they are making to hold onto their false belief, the healing effects will not last for very long as the source is still creating illness in its direction of influence. Also, even if an acupuncturist was trained in the way of moving the mind with the needles, which I believe is a rare and mostly lost form of acupuncture, the patient still must make the choice because nothing can influence the will in the mind to move if the patient has not chosen to do so.

Some balance to this last important point and some Exceptional situations; Divine influence as a mystery. Sometimes people are miraculously healed. The mind was somehow changed. I believe the Creator does not directly interfere with free will, so did the Creator help the person make the choice? I am not certain. But this can happen. It's a bit of a mystery. Another exceptional situation occurs in homeopathy. Sometimes (we do strive for always) the remedy is such a well-selected and perfectly matched mirror of Nature to the person's belief system, that by taking it, it seems that the belief is simply gone and the person is cured. I think on some level there is still choice and the remedy does not do the work *for* the patient, per se, but it can appear so. The healing and choice may take place in a deep sleep through the dreams. Another exceptional situation is in hands on healing when a healer moves the Qi and the emotions so well that a patient feels so good and happy that the belief no longer appears true in relation to the feeling and they therefore choose to let go of the belief spontaneously with the movement of Qi, the chakras, and the auric field.

When we do move into the level of the mind and release the

fundamental cause of illness, there is a tremendous amount of influence which is a quantum level more significant than even the healing that takes place on the emotional level. One slight change in the mind allows for an immense amount of healing energy to resume its flow and supply to the lower worlds of emotions and body.

The soul, in my opinion, remains untouched by the world. It does not mean that our soul is not moved by beauty, love, and other wondrous things. It also does not mean that we do not grow in our soul through our life's lessons. It means that it remains untouched by the corruption and wounding of the world. Its vibration is so high that it is beyond the influence of this world, in the same way that the mind is beyond the influence of body, because the body is too dense and is *Patiens*, to the mind and emotions. And yes, when we forget who we are and are mired in the false beliefs of the world, we do become disconnected from the *experience* of our soul to differing degrees, but it remains unscathed by our false choices. In my awareness, there is but one choice that can affect the soul. And that is the willful choice to sell one's soul for fame, fortune, and power.

Some balance about working with the body. Yes, we do not strictly address the disease at the physical body level. However, just as we discussed how exercising and moving the body can help move the dimension of emotions, when we are working with Holistic Counseling and other forms of healing that do address the fundamental cause of illness as it lives in the mind, it can also be helpful to combine adjunct therapies that help move some old stuckness in the body to accelerate the healing process. I've found using osteopathic manipulation to move the body, internal organs, and spine after Holistic Counseling and homeopathy, for instance, to be a very effective combination in certain cases of great stuckness in the body. Also, a chiropractic adjustment following some great release on the mental-emotional level can really bring about a hastened alignment of mind-emotion-body;

without these adjunct physical therapies, most of the time the body will align and begin to mirror the newly harmonious upper levels of the emotion and mind. It's just a matter of time. I've noticed my body adjusting to recent degrees of healing that have taken place in my awareness and emotion when I jog, or play hockey. I'll hear things popping into place. I'll feel muscles shifting to move vertebrae back in alignment. I will get a sense of the internal organs coming into a more open and aligned position. Once, I was playing hockey and I got tripped and fell onto my side on the hard ice. I was quite relaxed as I fell and when I hit the ice on my side, I heard a huge series of cavitations occurring along the length of my spine, as if I had had the most massive chiropractic adjustment right there on the spot. I saw a lot of lights and movement of Qi happened rapidly all over and within my body and my breathing changed to become much deeper and forceful for a few moments. When I got back onto my skates, I could breathe more deeply and I just felt great. I believe, in this way, Nature takes care of itself when the upper levels come more into alignment. The body will follow. When the body is very stuck, it is helpful to use some adjunct therapy and other forms of movement to facilitate the alignment of the dimensions of the whole person.

"Reich also noticed that as natural emotions were honestly expressed, movement and breathing also increased. Reich began working directly with movement and respiration in combination with psycho-emotional work. He also employed a unique form of massage to release the tension and memories stored in chronically contracted muscles."[6]

Male-Female – Finding the Balance (Important for Physician, Heal Thyself!)

In Holistic Counseling, it is essential for the practitioner to find a balance and harmony between their male and female energies. Regardless of sex, every human being is made up of male and female energies. Even within the four dimensions of the whole person, and the four elements, there exists male and female balances within each element and in each world. So, for instance, in regards to the soul's "gender", although it dwells in the world of Fire, which is *Agens*-Active-Father, the soul is also comprised of the balance with the female. The soul is therefore both male and female, just as the mind has both male and female traits. Willfulness is male, it is active. Observation and intuition are female. They are allowing. In the world of emotion, we see clear Yin-Yang, male-female principles in the chakras, the front being female, the rear being male, and in the body, we have Yin and Yang organs, as well as active elements of our autonomic nervous system (sympathetic) and passive (parasympathetic), as another example. When everything is boiled down to its very essence, that essence is a balance of male and female. Alchemy would say, Fire and Water. Father and Mother. *Agens* and *Patiens*. And in the Hermetic tradition, As Above, so Below. Another expression in alchemy is the "All in All."

Women tend to be naturally and more effortlessly inclined toward the female. Most societies allow and expect women to be more feminine. Men tend toward the male and are accepted and expected to be more so. But there are some women that are naturally far more masculine than many men tend to be, and some men that are very feminine in nature. So we cannot say men are male and women are female. It is also not accurate or true to state "Men are from Mars. Women are from Venus." It is a misconception that leaves us "half of ourselves," and also, codependent, needing the energy of the opposite sex to balance us.

The two closest and most influential planets to Earth are Mars and Venus. These were not placed in vain by the Creator. They represent and also literally influence the balance of life. When Mars and Venus work together in harmony, there is peace, there is protected love, there is strength, and there is health. When imbalances arise, disease and disharmony result. The other two most influential celestial orbs are the Sun and the Moon, equally balanced male-female counterparts. And isn't it a wonder to reflect on the fact that the Sun and Moon, although physically greatly different in size and influence, from Earth still appear to the human eye as being equal in size?

Everything in the world is made up of the balance of male and female, and Yin and Yang. Hot and cold. We have Yin organs and Yang organs. Day and night. Light and darkness. (Good and evil, however, are not the same sort of balance or counterparts as are male and female. Good and evil do not balance each other to bring about some greater whole. That is a common misconception and is something that is discussed at times during the course and that I address in my book on Kabbalah, *The Last Four Books of Moses*.) We have feeling centers and will centers. It is in finding the harmony between these two opposite – and sometimes seemingly *opposing* – energies that we achieve health in the mind, emotions, and body and peace on Earth. For the practitioner, finding this balance of Yin and Yang is an important part of 'Physician, Heal Thyself!'

In every class, I ask the students to list attributes of the male and female energies – both the positive traits, and the negative ones. The lists that we come up with are always very similar. Here is a table depicting many of the attributes of male and female.

MALE – YANG – MARS	FEMALE – YIN – VENUS
Positive Traits of Yang	Positive Traits of Yin
Active/Doing	Soft
Structure	Nurturing
Strong/Hard	Empathic/Caring/Sympathetic
Logic	Accepting
Organization	Creative
Linear	Intuitive

Vertical	Spherical
Warrior	Horizontal
Protective	Chaotic (as a positive aspect)
Boundaries	Passive
Saying No!	Vulnerable
Confidence	Yes! Doing for others
Outward	Inward
Goal oriented	Yielding
Fixer	Humble
Discernment	Giving
Focus	Sensitive
Provider	Selfless
Self-care	Vulnerable (as a positive aspect)
Seeing the negative	Seeing the Positive
Responsible	

Negative Traits of Yang

Aggressive
I'm the best – better than everyone else
Violent
Controlling
Forceful
War-mongering
Arrogance
Impatient
Know it all
Objectifying – sex
More shallow. On the surface
Selfish
Bullying

Negative Traits of Yin

Passive (as a negative trait)
Cutting oneself down "humility"/denial of greatness
Chaotic (as a negative trait)
Manipulative
Drama
Unprotected
Victim
Weak/lacking in power/decisiveness
Lack of confidence
Overly nurturing
Can't say no
Denial
Naive

When we look at the negative traits of each of the polar opposite energies, they are negative only because they are lacking in the balance of their opposite/counterpart. So when someone is too strong and assertive, it will be experienced as destructive and aggressive. They are too much in the Yang and not enough of the Yin gentleness to bring the strong assertiveness into balance. If someone cannot say no, it is because they lack the male sense of self to respect one's own boundaries. Selfishness, for example, is an important trait in a person's life. It is not all bad. It means to be thinking of self. However, if there is no thought of others, no concern or compassion for others, then that selfishness turns into a negative thing. One can only be too nurturing if one is not also nurturing the self. So it is really not possible to have too much of Yin or Yang. We can say that when one energy becomes more predominant, the other must rise up to bring harmony, or else the predominant energy becomes imbalanced and thus, negative.

In Holistic Counseling practice, and in Holism in general, problems arise with the imbalance of the practitioner being too much toward one direction or the other. Since Holistic Counseling is a non-directional practice, if the practitioner is too male, they will tend to try to control the outcome of the dialogue. They will think they know best and try to be energetically superior to the patient. They will also lack the warm, inviting compassion of the heart from the female energy and either intimidate the patient into answering questions or make them shut down altogether, out of a sense of feeling threatened, especially if that patient has issues around being dominated by the male energy (that has arisen from men in their lives, most likely, but also potentially from women as well). The too-male practitioner in Holistic Counseling will miss subtle intuitive promptings for a good question to ask, and will be too much up in their minds, not present with the emotional and intuitive information occurring in the healing space.

By contrast, a practitioner who is too female in nature will struggle with other issues in practice. They will tend to be too gentle and too soft, not asking the really tough questions that require the patient to take a good, hard, and oftentimes, painful look at themselves. The female energy is normally very intent on the well-being of the other, and has a struggle with confronting negativity, which is more an attribute that the male is capable of. So when a too-female practitioner encounters a place where a person does not want to go, they will yield and not keep up with the tough questions. Being very sensitive to the other's needs, a too-female practitioner will shy away from what they intuitively sense the patient does not wish to experience. Of course, no Holistic Counseling practitioner should ever push a person into a realm where they simply cannot go or will not go. But, in my practice, I often hit walls with patients, where, in the sick side of themselves, they have built up survival strategies. In essence, the illness has a life of its own and a strong will to live. The ego has also become intimately entangled in the illness. It is crucial for the male energy to be present, to discern this fact and know it is in the patient's best interest to confront and move through their illness and the ego that is attached to it. A lack of male energy in a too-female practitioner will get stuck at this point in the dialogue where some courage and toughness needs to be in the mix to bring a person through their tendency to want to avoid their problems and/or pretend that they don't have a problem.

Another issue encountered with too much female energy has to do with rescuing the person from their problems. As we work so closely with someone, it is easy to really take great pity on their suffering. The too-female energy tends to want to rescue and nurture the sick person by taking on their ills, rather than the male that allows the individual expression of the other to go through its own ordeal. "Oh, you poor thing. You need me to help you." (Unhealthy female) vs. "You're fine. You can go through this. You'll be ok." (More healthy male). This detachment that comes from the male energy is needed in practice. Everyone must ultimately make their own choices. That is very key in Holistic Counseling. If we care too much and become too meddlesome in the choices a person is making, that is actually not good for them. So even though the female energy wishes the best for the other, when it is out of balance, it is not good for the other person. On the other hand, having too little care and heartfelt emotion (too much male) for a person is also out of balance and will not bring enough fluidity and grace to one's practice. The practitioner must always review their state and seek to find the ever-so-subtle balance between Yin and Yang. I have found that where practitioners struggle the most is in embodying the sacred masculine energy. It seems that there is such a strong push toward the feminine in the healing and New Age world that the firmness, directness, and healthy boundaries that come along with the healthy male is missing or is too tentative and shy. Being the active element, the male energy's place in the balance is essential to be the most effective practitioner.

There is much that can be said about the balance of the male and female. In my teachings on Kabbalah, I go into much more depth and detail. I also explore more of this topic during the course. It is really quite simple, in essence. This doesn't mean that it is easy. It means it can be broken down to very basic principles that are not complicated. The application of the principles in life is where it can be quite challenging. What I suggest to you, the reader, now, at this point in the book is to always seek a balance and harmony between the male and the female that lives inside of you. Take a look at the table of attributes and think of what is second nature and where you are lacking or what seems like a very difficult struggle to embody. Then simply work on bringing more of the opposite to balance what you are used to being and doing. So if you tend to be very soft spoken and afraid of being too "arrogant," allow more assertiveness into your life. You are invited by the very make-up of the Universe around you to do so. The Universe, by its ubiquitous patterns of male and female attributes in the stars and planets, and in Nature Itself, has given each and everyone one of us the stamp of approval to embody both male and female energies.

If you tend to be very male and not very in touch with the emotional side of things, invite emotion, vulnerability, and openness into your life. By doing so, you do not lose the maleness. Inviting in the female does not erase or swallow up the male in a person. Also, do not fear bringing in too much of the opposite. It may seem that way, at first, because it is so foreign and so opposite to what one is used to. But really, when a person is very well established in one side of the polarities, there is little risk of them ever getting out of balance by inviting in the opposite. They will simply learn to become a blend of the two polarities. So it is with physicians healing themselves.

More on the Mind-Body Connection

We often use the term, mind-body connection, and it is a bit of a misnomer, because it would more accurately be mind-emotion-body connection. However, we will keep in mind that when the term mind-body connection is used, that there is a watery medium that helps achieve this connection. One of my favorite areas of understanding is to recognize how the mind and body are connected. What is nice to be able to piece together is how this comes about. In the last section, we discussed how every-thing is comprised of a balance of male and female. This will help us recognize the dynamics of the mind-body connection and also, how the mind is at the root cause, that is, the fundamental cause of chronic disease.

In Traditional Chinese Medicine (TCM) the Yin/Female organs create the precious substance that nourishes the body, and the Yang organs are responsible for the active part of using, spreading, burning, and distributing the precious substance created by the Yin organ. We can say that the Yin organs receive the life force energy in the form of Qi and create the precious substance passively, through this receptivity. In this way, at the level of the organs, the male or Yang energy is somewhat secondary to the Yin organ, which is primary and source of the precious substance. This is true as well for the chakra system. In TCM, the front of the body is Yin and the back of the body is Yang. This also corresponds with Barbara Brennan's teaching on the chakras – that the front chakras are receptive, and afferent in

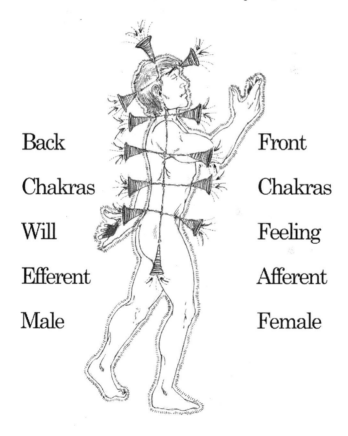

Back

Chakras

Will

Efferent

Male

Front

Chakras

Feeling

Afferent

Female

nature.[7] They are the feeling centers. Afferent and receptive is passive. This is the essence of the female. And the rear chakras are the will, efferent centers, which is male. This helps us gain an even deeper understanding as to the workings of our whole person. The precious substance, the precious life force from The Healing Power of Nature and the Universe is received by the female. The male energy is the active part which wills, directs or simply works in harmony with this source of vital life energy.

Barbara Brennan also states, "The powerful flow of life force that comes with the involuntary divine creative principle cannot be commanded by the ego. Another way to say this is that the goodness within you flows of its own accord; it reaches out in wisdom, love, and caring of its own accord. It does not flow on the command of the ego. The only thing the ego can do is stop it from flowing or get out of its way."[8]

This quote describes a principle that very appropriately applies to the functioning of the front and rear chakras. They are normally naturally open and receptive and flowing in harmony with the Universal life force. Here we can understand a little more about The Healing Power of Nature. When all is well, the front chakras are open and are naturally receiving The Healing Power of Nature. Like funnels of energy, the front, feeling chakras receive energy from Nature and distribute it into their corresponding organs, areas, and acupuncture meridians. So, for instance, the third/solar plexus chakra receives energy and distributes it to the liver, gallbladder, spleen, stomach, pancreas, as well as the intestines, the muscles, bones, skin, and nerves also in this area. The energy is also distributed along the acupuncture meridians corresponding to the mentioned organs, directly from the chakra. First the Qi flows into the meridians, and then into the organs. This makes sense since the meridians are needled in acupuncture order to restore balance to the organs, and not vice versa. When all is well, the reception of life force energy and its flow through the body is uninhibited and the organs, meridians and corresponding body parts are nourished with Nature's ever-present healing power. It is when the ego gets in the way, as suggested by Barbara Ann Brennan's quote just above, that the trouble begins.

But how does the ego get in the way, and why?

First of all, let's have a look at the rear, will chakras. These will chakras are efferent in nature. Meaning, we can carry out an active will through these centers. The rational mind is the part of our mind that carries out this will-based function. When the flow of life force is uninhibited, the rear-will centers are in "allow" mode – which is essentially doing nothing besides simply allowing the front, afferent chakras to receive the precious energy from the Universe. Or, we can say, they are working in the same direction, carrying out a will that is harmonious with the flow of the receptive, source, Yin chakras, like a person lying on their stomach on a surfboard, riding a wave while also using their arms to push in the same direction. I imagine that the rear, will chakras are also involved in the distribution and direction of healthy life force to the corresponding areas of the body just as the Yang organs distribute and use the precious Qi generated in the Yin organs.

Now let's imagine the following scenario. Little Tina is playing in the sandbox with some friends.

She, for some reason, is slow in developing her voice and her expression is quiet and shy. At times, she has a hard time pronouncing words. Her friends notice this. One of her friends, a leader, notices this and makes fun of her and says, "Are you stupid or something?" The rest of the children laugh. Even though the leader's words are not necessarily intended to be hurtful, Tina feels crushed. Children have very keen imaginations and even the smallest comments can be interpreted in a very creative imaginative way and can have lifelong impact on a person's well-being. This particular sort of idea would zero right in on the third chakra, which has to do with one's self-esteem and a sense of belonging. With any offensive attack or criticism of this nature, we all have a choice of whether or not to believe it, but Little Tina, being so young, is like most children, and has little defense against this. She will allow this comment to enter past her protective boundary (this protective boundary is a healthy aspect of the mind that is male in nature and is responsible for 'guarding' one's inner world against untrue thoughts and 'accusations') and she receives an energetic "punch" in the third chakra area. This energetic hit doesn't feel very good for Tina and she will do as most humans do – try to stop herself from feeling any of it.

There are many things people do externally to avoid feeling pain and other unpleasant emotions and feelings like fear, anxiety, self-loathing, despair, etc. People drink. They eat chocolate and comfort food. They do drugs. They work too hard. Exercise too much. Watch too much television. All to avoid uncomfortable feelings. The most primal way suppression occurs is via the rear, will chakra. Little Tina doesn't like how the energy in the third chakra area feels so unpleasant and uncomfortable. So she will subconsciously, or very subtly on the conscious level, say to herself; "This feeling is bad. I don't want to feel it." And just like that, the rational mind gives the command to the will center in the back of the third chakra to not feel. It's like the will center clamps down on the flow, trying to stop it, like squeezing a hose to stop the flow of water. This is also similar to the way a person will grasp and tighten their muscles around an injury, in an attempt to stop feeling the pain of the trauma. What also occurs as a consequence to a person using their will to stop the flow is that it disconnects them from the feeling of the naturally incoming energy of the front aspect of the chakra. This disconnect is common following mental-emotional trauma. In order to not feel, the person needs to continue to be in control, because if they stop controlling, then the flow returns, which brings back the pain. What a person really wants to do in order to feel ok again is to allow the pain to be felt. It won't last forever, and then the natural and healthy feeling is restored to the corresponding chakra. The Healing Power of Nature is ever ready, waiting to be allowed to flow, to bring the flow of the Universal life force back into the body. With a healthy third chakra, that feeling is a sense of belonging, confidence in oneself, "I am ok." The surrounding organs, muscles, and other tissues are supplied with the Universal life energy/Qi. When a trauma enters the picture that resonates at the level of a certain chakra (confidence at the third chakra, love for others at the fourth chakra, expression at the fifth chakra, etc.) and the person blocks it using their rational mind via the rear, will chakra, they are not able to discernibly block the "bad" feeling and allow the good feeling. All flow gets shut down and the Universal life force is blocked in that area. The surrounding vital organs and tissues will not get their proper nourishing flow and dis-ease will settle into one of the areas. In the third chakra, for instance, it can express itself with stomach aches. Ulcers. Indigestion. Heartburn. Back pain in the area. Muscular tension. Subluxations. Nerve pain. And much more serious illness as well.

This is one way of understanding how a certain belief and emotional trauma results in disease. The wound begins in the mind. Specifically, it has to do with choosing a false and harmful idea, which is not in harmony with our I AM statement, as being true. The false belief enters into the mental sphere by allowing it/choosing it/identifying with it as true, when it really is not in harmony with the well-being of a person. Since the idea is untrue, it has ill effects in one's system, just as putting the wrong sort of fuel in a certain engine will cause it to malfunction. "Wrongful" or incorrect thoughts are like plugs to the true state of the being. *Because* a thought is not true, *we have to* hold onto it with our will, otherwise, if we didn't, it would drift away and be gone simply by the fact that it is not true and thus, holds no substance in reality. This is why I recommend the following thought experiment for healing. "Everything we know, or think we know, we must let go of." If something is true, it will return.

If it is not true, it will be gone and not return. This liberates us from the false belief by not having to carry it and also, beautifully, it reveals a most important fact about what is true about ourselves and that is: If we let go of a belief about ourselves and it returns, (for e.g. – I am a good person), then we see it is not us that is *responsible* for the creation of the truth. It is simply an observation of a fact about our nature. In other words, this supports the fact that we didn't create ourselves nor our I AM statement! Our Creator has granted us with that most priceless gift of life and existence. (Yes, we are involved, in a very spiritual "before we manifested in this life" sort of way, in creating ourselves where we co-exist as One with the Creator. But for understanding once we have manifested in this world in this life, we are not responsible for this level of creation.) So, when we let go of the control over our thoughts, we then re-attune with The Healing Power of Nature by observing who we are (female) and then we know who we are (male) by the observation. This helps us become more humble and accept that we do not need to hold onto what is true about ourselves, but rather, observe and accept (female) and then understand and act on it (male).

Be – Do
Accept – Act
Feel – Follow

With a false belief in the mind and action of the will to hold this false premise in the rear chakra, the emotional feeling happens in a secondary fashion following the false thoughts. "I am stupid" resonates with the third chakra area, since the third chakra deals with a sense of self-confidence. It is like throwing a wrench into a properly functioning motor. This gets in the way of the normal good feelings of the third chakra (I feel good about myself) and results in an unpleasant feeling (I am not so good, I am stupid). Subsequently, this unpleasant feeling is then equally judged as bad and the rational mind uses the rear will center to further block the flow. As a person goes through life, the false belief that was chosen (I am stupid) results in a very unpleasant feeling in the third chakra area. It feels insecure, it feels shut down where it should/could normally feel confident, good in one's own skin. So while a person is undergoing healing, both the false belief and the subsequent painful emotion needs to be addressed.

Later in life, Little Tina grows up and sees a Holistic Counselor. She could use a little healing. She has experienced difficulties in the realm of self-confidence her entire life. She has had digestive issues and chronic fatigue, due to her constantly pushing herself to prove to others and herself that she is not stupid (this is part of the *Two Paths and Compensation* that I speak about later). Via a process of engaging her in simple, yet ever deeper questions, she arrives at both the painful difficult feelings as well as the actual belief itself. In certain cases, just by recognizing the belief itself is no longer true (and ultimately, never was), the healthy, natural emotional flow is re-established because it was always held back by the core belief. One feels returned to their true, healthy state by having released the core false belief. The Universal life force resupplies the true sense of "I am ok". The waters just flow back in when the dam is removed. In other cases, the patient must be encouraged to allow themselves to feel the pain that arises as they contact the root of their problem. Since the pain of the original wound is what many people try to avoid, anything which threatens to bring this to light and to be dealt with may be avoided like the plague, and that includes healing. This is where the practitioner has to reassure the patient of what is happening and give supportive explanations about how this is the direction they truly wish to go in to re-establish the healthy flow of their life force and lead the life they have been yearning to live. Allowing the feeling reconnects with the flow, and moves the old, painful energies through their system to return to a sense of goodness in the affected area.

At times, even while letting go of a false belief system, without allowing oneself to feel the pain that has been suppressed for a long time, the emotions can remain blocked, which makes it very difficult to re-establish the idea of being alright because one does not feel alright. Because one does not feel ok, or good about themselves, it is easy to reconnect with the thought in the mind of not being ok, of being stupid. It's like the unhealthy emotion cries out for its false belief system counterpart, like the sick Eve reaching out to the sick Adam. So Little Tina, now older and in Holistic Counseling says yes, now I do recognize that I am not stupid and I choose to release this idea from my mind, but I still feel very lacking in confidence in myself. Out of habit, she has continued to resist the flow of her third chakra, to avoid feeling that original wound. She has created a sort of emotional monster from the belief system. So even though her mind begins to grasp that she is not stupid as she has believed, the emotional energy is blocked in her third chakra, which feels like a lack of confidence (since confidence is the normal, healthy state of that chakra). This is why the emotional feeling of a wound must also be allowed to be contacted and felt without judgment (and also to not regard it as truth, but as the reflection of what the belief was that gave rise to it) in order for the true and healthy direction and flow of the feeling to be re-established. Healing Power of Nature re-enter!

A belief system, even a false one, can be something someone becomes invested in. In other words, they feel they *have* to believe it, their life depends on it, it supports them, it makes them feel better. It helps them avoid dealing with the actual pain of their existence. For example, 'I am better than others.' This is not an uncommon form of belief for people who have low self-esteem and have been put down, mostly by one of their parents, and made to feel inferior. The belief system is a way of surviving by overcompensating for the feeling of being inferior. A person who has chosen to believe they are better than others will seek to prove that to themselves and others, by putting others down, just as their parents did to them. When they "prove it," it makes them feel better. It's like the negative space of their wounded self that feels inferior becomes a little hungry monster that feeds off the putting down of others. So as the belief "I am better" that was adopted in order to survive the even deeper wound of believing "I am inferior to others" is uncovered in the Holistic Counseling Dialogue, it will not want to let go until the deeper belief "I am inferior" is also unearthed and released. When the deeper belief is explored and the choice to hold onto that is revealed and then released, all other beliefs that have grown out of it will have no more rootedness to survive. In simple terms, it is no longer needed. This is an insight into the *"House of Cards"* metaphor which will be examined further later.

Chapter 5

To Heal Each Person as an Individual

This is a very simple principle. If we have 100 people with migraines, each person has a different root cause that led to their migraines. For one, it is constant worry that they won't be able to make ends meet. For another, it is the suppression of their sexual energy. And yet for another, the migraines occur as a manifestation of the person overworking their mind in order to appear highly intelligent to compensate for a feeling of insecurity or worthlessness. For another, they feel so under pressure in their life that the head manifests the same pressure they are feeling placed under in their life.

In my years of specializing in myasthenia gravis, I've yet to see two cases alike. I have, from time to time, recognized similar elements between two cases, and I do observe some form of harsh attack or self-criticism that a person perpetrates on themselves (which is common in auto-immune disease), but never have the root causes been exactly the same in two cases of myasthenia gravis. So even though one knows that in auto-immune diseases, for instance, there is a root of attacking the self mentally and emotionally which is reflected by the immune system turning against the self, this doesn't really help much beyond being a guiding light to get to the specific and *unique way* in which that *individual* is attacking themselves. Imagine developing a product that would advertise to help the auto-immune sufferer, "Stop Attacking Yourself!" The modern world and business enterprises are always trying to mass produce things, making them widespread and accessible to a large number of people for optimal profits. This does not work for true Holism as it removes working with each person as an individual – again, a true and important principle of our medicine. Each case must be addressed by having an attitude of discovery rather than knowing. Nature is ever creative and the lover of Nature and healing must be ever ready to see what is there rather than project what one thinks they know.

Chapter 6

Doctor as Teacher

The greatest good you can do for another is not just share your riches, but reveal to them their own.
Benjamin Disraeli

When a person undergoing Holistic Counseling treatment has an "aha" moment, what better way can a doctor act as teacher, than to simply provide the space to bring about the learning about the truth of their nature. A doctor can say, "Drink more water. Get better exercise. Eat these healthy foods." And this definitely does fulfill *doctor as teacher* as well. But nothing compares to the teaching a doctor facilitates inside of the person when they discover an unmistakable truth by the process of answering questions directed at themselves. It is the highest form of *doctor as teacher*. Also in homeopathy, as well as in all true holistic medicines, a lot of learning comes about through the healing that the remedy or healing itself brings. People spontaneously begin to understand things about themselves and about the Nature of the world that remained veiled to them earlier. A doctor can attempt to offer this form of teaching to a patient that is veiled, through advice, instruction, but it will not be able to penetrate. And the doctor is really just tooting their own horn. It will be in one ear of the patient and out the other, or it will not make sense on a core level to bring about any useful action. Only when the Vital Force moves and/or the root of the problem that blocks the patient from "seeing the light" is removed can the true teaching take effect. Then we fulfill *doctor as teacher* in the most profound sense.

People tend to try everything *but* face what they need to understand about themselves that has led to their illness. They try all the therapies out there. All the supplements. The latest fads. The newest diets. Nothing helps in a lasting fashion. None of those practitioners asked the important question, "*What is really troubling you?*" No one helped them connect what is going on in their body with what is going on in their lives at large, as well as in the subtler dimensions of their being. When I am referred a patient, or a patient comes to me from another practitioner, I am often surprised at how little the other practitioner did to investigate the person's struggles, their pain, their false ideas that are causing suffering. It's like practitioners are afraid or don't know how to peel back the thin veil that sits between the outer presentation of ourselves and our symptoms and the inner workings of ourselves. This veil is so widely held in our modern society and so rarely addressed and traversed. It's like the practitioner is afraid to violate that private space. I ask you this: Is it a violation to gently ask people questions to get them to think and come up with answers to their deepest struggles? If, by walking with a person through the jungle of their subconscious, you help them arrive at a place of peace and health, has anything wrong been perpetrated? Is anything violated? The answer to these questions is no and the more a practitioner has healed themselves and others through this deep investigative method seen in Holistic Counseling, the more clear this becomes. Truly, it simply is a matter of fact. Of course, permission must always be acquired before engaging in such a personal and deep exploration. This normally comes easily because the patient is seeking help and they have come to you, the practitioner, because you can help them. Patients really respect and easily work in accordance with a practitioner's knowing of the direction that needs to be followed that will bring about their healing and relief from suffering. This is different from a doctor telling a patient what to do. It is a doctor having trust and faith to guide the patient through the process that will be of the greatest benefit for them. This is something good that patients can then also trust in. This is also one of the very few ways in which a doctor can use the power that comes with that office to guide the patient in the direction they need to follow.

Chapter 7

Physician, Heal Thyself!

In my book, *The Revolution of Naturopathic Medicine*, I introduced the 7th principle of Naturopathic philosophy, which was missing in our philosophy. It is of utmost importance in keeping with holistic practice. As I described in the introduction, one cannot practice holistically if one has not begun the process of healing themselves. It doesn't take perfection. There is not an "arrival point" of health or well-being that marks the place where one can begin working with others. But that initiation onto the path of self-healing must begin before one launches into holistic healing to help others. If this path has not begun for the practitioner, the knowing and experience of healing from personal experience is lacking. So when one encounters the pressure in practice that exists because a patient is confronting their wounds and pain, it is almost inevitable that a practitioner will make the easy choice toward an allopathic prescription. Without having made their own better choices for healing, a practitioner will turn away from helping to guide a person into understanding their root cause of illness. They in turn will not select a path that is healthier and truer to the patient. When one has gone through their own pain and has found the great reward in health and vitality as a result, there is no question about the benefit that comes from facing the darkness inside of ourselves. This becomes the incentive and even the faith in knowing the person is going in the right direction as they step into the outer boundaries of the dark forest of their subconscious.

Chapter 8

The Three Models of Medicine with Principles Checklist

The Three Models of Practicing Medicine are Allopathic, Systems-based, and Holistic. This is something that I first published in my book *The Revolution of Naturopathic Medicine*. The ideas themselves are not so much new and originally from me, except for the idea of NDs practicing 'Systems-based' medicine. I am simply illustrating some important points to bring the principles of Naturopathic and real Holistic medicine into perspective. Let's take a look at the three models of the practice of medicine and then determine which principles of the philosophy of Holism and Naturopathy are applied for each medicine.

The Allopathic Model

We'll start with the allopathic model since it is the most pervasive model practiced in medicine throughout the planet. I dare say, sadly enough, up until the day this book is published, it is even the most practiced model within Naturopathic medicine. Evidence-based medicine is quite allopathic in nature. It tends to take itself very seriously. That is partly necessary because of safety first – do no harm. The rest is getting lost in the minutiae of actions and interactions on the level of the body and how to combat the symptoms of disease.

The trend of modern medical research and practice in our great colleges and endowed research institutes is almost entirely along combative lines. Henry Lindlahr (1862 – 1924)

The allopathic model is simple enough to grasp.
The body is considered a machine. (Mechanistic model.)

When a part has a problem (is sick), you fix the part through drugs, supplements, herbs, or surgery. It's a this-for-that medicine. There's a pill for every ill. Or a supplement for every ailment. We all have heard the first expression. I made that second one up, since it seems to be true for "evidence based" allopathic Naturopathy and since the pharmaceutical companies are moving into the Nutraceutical industry, we'll be seeing more "natural" supplements for more ailments:

For hypertension – a hypotensive agent.
For constipation – a laxative.
For a skin condition – something that clears up the skin.

The idea is also that if a part has a problem it is defective and needs help to function. Without this drug or supplement, your body part will never recover. It cannot heal on its own. That is the idea behind the allopathic model. In most cases of chronic illness, that is not true. In some extreme situations, there is not the luxury of time to allow for the part to be healed holistically. In such a case, we need the allopathic model.

When people at dinner parties hear that I am a Naturopathic doctor, they ask me questions like, "What's good for migraines?" Or, "What do you give for constipation?" Or any number of different conditions, equally of a mental or emotional nature, like anxiety, depression, or bipolar. It's then that I give my little, "I don't treat conditions. Rather, I work with each person individually and look for the root cause of the disease as it lives in the mental-emotional sphere, and that is always different for each person." Depending on where I am, but more often than not, this usually ends the conversation and leaves people looking disappointed and glossy-eyed. However, sometimes, people are interested to know what that means, and some state that they agree and see it that way as well, and that is a good day indeed.

It is necessary at times to treat allopathically, and when doing so, it is best to have a clear diagnosis of the problem, good knowledge of biomedical science, and also good research and knowledge of the different 'things' we can offer for the conditions requiring allopathic treatment. Because it is a form of medicine that works on the physical plane, through the body, it's important to be well educated regarding harmful interactions between drugs and when certain drugs, herbs, and supplements are contraindicated. In other words, mindfulness and carefulness are important so that we *do no harm*.

Here are some of the main examples of conditions requiring allopathic treatment:

Emergencies (ER).
Very Acute forms of disease.
Critical care.
Extreme life-threatening forms of illness.
Surgeries. Orthopedic injuries.
The very elderly. Severely mentally impaired.

For some of these, we can still use homeopathy, which, when taking into account the whole symptom picture, tends to be an essentially Holistic medicine. But if we're unable to do homeopathy, these conditions can require an allopathic approach. The most important message here is that – if someone is greatly and acutely suffering, and if their life is at risk, then we must save the life, before we do anything else. The soul affects the mind. The mind affects the emotions. The emotions affect the body. When the body is affected, it leads towards death. When the body is so severely affected and time is of the essence, we want to control and slow or stop the progress toward death. That is done at the level of the body and is one of the good purposes of allopathic medicine. Life is precious.

I believe eventually computers will be the allopaths of the

future. You will go to a machine, stick your head in the machine. The machine will scan your face, your sclera, your irises, and look into your retina. It will take your blood pressure and heart rate. It will pluck a sample of your hair. It will have you breathe into a sensor to read the gasses of your breath. It will take a drop of blood. It may even have you pee in a little cup. Then, within a few moments, it will finish scanning all the possible known conditions you have, and will spit out a prescription for the drugs or supplements best known to treat that condition. All the more reason to learn how to practice holistically. Keep your job.

Principles Checklist for the Allopathic Model

√ First of all, to do no harm.
• To heal the whole person
• To act in cooperation with The Healing Power of Nature.
• To address the fundamental cause of disease.
• To heal each person as an individual
• Doctor as Teacher
• Physician, Heal Thyself! (ie. does an allopathic doctor need to heal themselves to be effective?)

In this exercise, I endeavored to be as generous as I could. I gave a little checkmark for doing no harm, provided we practice responsibly, knowing the right doses, indications, contraindications, interactions and everything else that we need to consider when applying this model of medicine. However, it is not entirely true that allopathic treatment does no harm. As discussed earlier, when a symptom is suppressed, as in the metaphor of the crying child, it creates a worsening in the mistunement of the Vital Force. This is a form of harm. When life is not at risk, then we do not need to use the allopathic approach, except in some rare situations that call for it, which I discuss later in this book.

The System-Based Model

As the title of this method of medicine implies, the systems-based model of medicine involves the direct treatment of the various systems in the body. We have many systems.

Central Nervous. Immune. Circulatory. Respiratory. Digestive. Endocrine. Sexual. Elimination. Dental. Dermatological, etc.

And on more subtle levels – Acupuncture system of meridians. Chakras. Auric field.

The idea in the systems-based approach is that health ensues when we have healthy functioning systems.

The key to health, is having a healthy gut. So we've got to eliminate leaky gut syndrome. Move the bowels and eliminate constipation. Good nutrition.

The key to health is having a healthy liver. Detox and support the liver! (Naturopaths love detoxing the liver.)

The key to health is having a strong immune system. Support and strengthen the immune system.

Chiropractic. The key to health lies in having a healthy, aligned spine free of subluxations. Chiropractors even go to some length to claim that the cause of illness lies in an unhealthy spine. Solution – adjust the spine.

Following the systems-based approach, a practitioner can help a patient feel much better. There's no doubt about it. Being detoxified, moving the bowels better, having an aligned spine will all promote a better sense of health. In acupuncture, the goal is to restore balance to the meridian and organ system. Even in subtle healing modalities, like Reiki and hands on healing, we work to restore balance and correct disharmonies and blockages in the energetic field and the chakra system.

But what of the whole person? How holistic is this? And in the long run, how much are we really helping our patients by only practicing the systems-based model of medicine? I have spoken to chiropractors who recognize that the subluxations they are correcting keep returning and the causes of the problems need to be addressed deeper to prevent this return. Also, when we keep the gut functioning healthily, *only* on the level of the gut, what if the body wishes to express some form of problem that is a reflection of a deeper issue? When we keep the problem corrected only at the level of the system, we do create some "back pressure" at the deeper level and worsen the Vital Force mistunement.

Principles Checklist for the Systems-Based Model
√ • First of all, to do no harm.
   • To heal the whole person
√ • To act in cooperation with The Healing Power of Nature.
   • To address the fundamental cause of disease.
√ • To heal each person as an individual
√ • Doctor as Teacher
√ • Physician, Heal Thyself!

In this exercise as well, I endeavored to be as generous as I could.

I gave a small checkmark because we can practice consciously, mindfully, and carefully and do no harm.

We are acting, in a small way in cooperation with The Healing Power of Nature, by eliminating toxins, restoring alignments, balancing systems, allowing more Qi to flow and restoring balance, so a small check mark is given for that. In some cases, we may be addressing the fundamental cause of disease if the disease has been elicited through the diet, through toxicity, and as a result of strictly environmental factors. It is true that we are moving into the functioning of systems, which is deeper than prescribing for outward symptoms, but it's not worthy of giving a check mark for addressing the fundamental cause, because the fundamental cause is usually much deeper. We are working with each person as an individual, to determine which system is most out of balance, so I gave that a medium sized check mark. And a medium sized checkmark is also generously awarded to Doctor as teacher, because a practitioner has the opportunity to impart a lot of helpful knowledge to the patient regarding lifestyle, nutrition, exercise, etc. For the most part, a physician does not need to heal themselves to do systems-based work, but can remain emotionally shut down and removed during the practice, except in more subtle energetic medicines like acupuncture, Reiki and hands on healing, where the practitioner's own Vital Force energy is involved in the healing. So for that, a small check mark was awarded.

The Holistic Model

Ultimately, the entire universe has to be understood as a single, undivided whole, in which analysis into separately and independently existent parts has no fundamental status.
David Bohm (1917 – 1992)

The definition of holistic:
"ho·lis·tic /hōΑlistik/
1. Characterized by comprehension of the parts of something as intimately interconnected and explicable only by reference to the whole."[9]

Whereas the allopathic model and even systems-based model address the parts of the whole as separate individual parts or systems, the Holistic model understands that each part is a representation and is intimately interconnected to the whole. So when there is disease or a problem in a part or in a system, it is only because the part is manifesting the problem that exists on the whole. And when we say the whole, it means the whole person. This means that there is a problem also existing in the mind; the emotions and the body are all an expression of that. The body is the final and densest "gateway" for the expression of the problem.

I'd like to clarify an error that is often made by people, both naturopath and lay alike, when discussing Holistic medicine and what it means. The terms Holism and holistic are largely misused today. I have seen labels for holistic toothpaste and holistic hair products in health food stores. Other times, someone feels they are practicing holistically because they give a herb for the pain in someone's joints, prescribe good diet for their nutrition, meditation exercises for the patient's mind, and a Bach flower remedy for the person's emotions. This approach is not unifying in nature. It does not help to connect the mind and the body and remains largely disjointed, which is, in essence, the opposite of Holism. Where is there a thread that unites mind and body? Are all of the principles of Naturopathic medicine being embraced? Is the fundamental cause of illness being addressed? Where is the connection between the manifestation of symptoms in the body and their source in the mind? For something to be (w)holistic, the WHOLE person must be looked at in such a way that there is not a separation between what a patient experiences in their physical symptoms and their mental-emotional spheres. To have a true Holism, our medicine must apply the principles of the philosophy of Naturopathic medicine altogether, as a whole, because it is a philosophy that extends beyond just Naturopathic medicine. It is the philosophy of Holism itself.

I have often marvelled at how the whole has been found represented on just about every part of the physical body. The face, ear, abdomen, and tongue, for instance, as exemplified through Traditional Chinese Medicine, all carry signatures of the whole, so that one can treat and/or diagnose through each of the small parts. One can needle, for instance, the liver, through a point on the ear. One can see a discoloration around the eyes on the face which points to a liver imbalance. One can palpate the abdomen at a specific point to test for tenderness, pain, or discomfort that also points to an issue with the liver and other organs of the body. Equally, one can look at the iris, in Iridology, or the sclera, in Sclerology, to diagnose issues anywhere in the body. The entire body can be diagnosed and treated through the sole of the foot, in Reflexology. With the whole being imprinted in so many parts, it calls forth the idea that every part must have the map of the whole.

What Holism really teaches us is that any part, like with these examples, but also with literally any part, including the pinky toe, or even a cell in the pinky toe, is intimately connected with the whole. One can extrapolate issues that are happening on the whole by comprehending the expression of the issue in the part. In Chapter 30 on *Technique of going through the Physical Symptoms to Get to the Root Cause*, I explain how to get to understand the root cause of the illness by going through the physical symptoms. It's like putting a mental-emotional stethoscope to the part to "listen" to what it is saying about the problem with the whole.

The Holistic model is the basis for this book, for this technique, and for all healing that occurs that is lasting, deep, and that positively impacts not just the person's health, but their entire life and their relationship with the world and with Nature.

The 6 principles of the Naturopathic philosophy are an illustration of Holism. When one applies the points of philosophy in practice, one is working holistically. This way of delineating the philosophy of Naturopathic medicine was not chosen in vain. It is in this fashion that one can most help a sick person because applying these principles is actually working the most in cooperation and harmony with The Healing Power of Nature.

Principles Checklist for the Holistic Model

√ • First of all, to do no harm.
√ • To heal the whole person
√ • To act in cooperation with The Healing Power of Nature.
√ • To address the fundamental cause of disease.
√ • To heal each person as an individual

√ • Doctor as Teacher
√ • Physician, Heal Thyself!

Holistic Counseling is actually one of the only modalities or methods of treatment that embodies all the principles of the entire philosophy of Naturopathic medicine. By asking questions to get to the root cause of illness, we address and remove the fundamental cause of illness and allow The Healing Power of Nature to enter therein. We are also working with each person as an individual, regardless of the illness they may be suffering from. Each illness lives differently in each person and many have different causes. Even though I have discovered there is a theme of a person being very hard and attacking themselves in auto-immune diseases, the way in which they do this, the language they use, the intensity, the fashion, is different for every individual. I really have seen no two cases of myasthenia gravis that are alike in all the years I've been practicing. As I begin to ask questions surrounding a person's life and what led to their illness, a rich, unique landscape unfolds during the dialogue. It is fascinating and truly is a privilege to help a person unravel the mystery of their struggles.

In Holistic Counseling, we also work with the whole person, the principle in Naturopathic medicine which most directly nods in acknowledgment of Holism. More importantly, in Holistic Counseling we establish a connection between the mind, emotions, and body of a person and do not work with the different dimensions of a person in a disjointed fashion. There is a beauty in the precision of isolating the thread that runs through a person's life that led to their illness. It gathers everything up into the healing process and leaves a person with a simple truth to acknowledge and let go of, rather than a piecemeal method of giving something for the mind, something for the emotions, and something for the body. A well-applied session of Holistic Counseling should leave the person understanding how a certain unhealthy belief they've been carrying became expressed in their body as the physical symptoms they are struggling with. A person who struggles with chronic migraines needs some investigation to the root cause of the migraines. This is the gift of the mind-body connection, where a person, through their own process, discovers what is underlying their illness. After this experience, a person can never look the same at the world. They can never go back to ignoring the signs the body is communicating from the disturbance in the Vital Force. They have an insight into Nature itself and how they were living out of harmony with it. They have, in short, become a better person through the process of their disease.

And in holistic practice, we must be physicians who are working on ourselves or else all the rest of the philosophy grinds to a halt and becomes fancy concepts rather than applicable principles.

In Holism, we see a thread extend across the person's life. The phrase I often share in class, "How someone does anything is how they do everything" applies largely to this holistic perspective. When I am in a "state", as I call it, meaning I am dealing with some issues, I can see the issues manifesting as stress, conflict, or trouble across the board in my life. For instance, at times, I have gotten into an issue of lacking confidence in myself. I will sense a hesitation in myself when selecting remedies for my patients. It's like I am holding back from allowing myself to trust my instincts. I experience the same issue on the ultimate Frisbee field in regards to making certain throws. I will have a difficult throw that ordinarily I could make without too much trouble, yet when I feel that lack of trust in myself to make it, I will hold back and choose another, "safer" or more certain throw. Underlying this holding back and hesitation is a fear of making mistakes. And what happens if I were to make a mistake? Well, funny you should ask. It would mean I am not perfect. And there you have the underlying cause, in my own case, manifesting as issues across the board, as a thread that, as in a fabric, weaves across a person's life and unites elements of the life where the same issue is manifesting.

In Holism, we do not separate between how a person lives, breathes, thinks, works, makes friends, makes love, fathers, mothers, goes to sleep, eats, sings, dances, or plays games. We see the Vital Force expressing itself, in essence, through every action. Surely, there are some areas of a person's life where they are not threatened in their insecurities and fears. But in all areas of a person's life where there is a perceived threat to their wounds, they will react in a typical way that is unique to them. For instance, if someone had the trauma of being left out of a group, be it their friends or their family, in any situation where they may potentially be left out, they will react with some form of control, or fear reaction, which leads them on a path of disease. If such a person is placed in a situation where there is no threat to their fear, they will not experience any of their pathology or need to respond with control to avoid experiencing their fear. So it is truly up to the practitioner of Holistic Counseling to be as a "detective of Nature" to find the thread and see it to its lowest denominator, that is, to its root. I find the metaphor of "Going down the Rabbit Hole" to be very appropriate in Holistic Counseling.

Chapter 9

The Vital Force – Implications for Holistic Counseling

From Hahnemann's Organon:

> In the healthy human state, the spirit-like life force (autocracy) that enlivens the material organism as "dynamis," governs without restriction and keeps all parts of the organism in admirable, harmonious, vital operation, as regards both feelings and functions, so that our indwelling rational spirit can freely avail itself of this living, healthy instrument for the higher purpose of our existence.[10]

I am truly grateful to have learned homeopathy. I have such a profound love and respect for this most powerful of medicines. I do not think I would be as good a practitioner of Holistic Counseling, nor have such an understanding of the workings of the mind, if I did not study homeopathy and learn the philosophies in Hahnemann's *Organon*. It is a bit of a shame that the *Organon* is not studied by all practitioners of medicine, be them conventional doctors, counselors, therapists, Naturopathic doctors and other alternative health practitioners. Because the philosophy in the *Organon* is part of the discipline of Homeopathy, people don't read it if they are not studying or practicing Homeopathy, although it is really full of Universal truths and principles of healing in medicine that all people should understand when dealing with health. It is not for nothing that those who oppose Vitalism and Holism in general in Naturopathic medicine also normally have a vehement opposition to homeopathy.

The first main important area to better understand Holism from the perspective of homeopathy and the *Organon* that I'd like to share relates to the understanding of the Vital Force that lives in each of us and how it responds to external and internal stimuli. Naturopathic doctors, independent of homeopathy, also have an equivalent recognition of this Vital Force, which they have called "The vital principle" or simply "Vitalism."

The Vital Force is our inner energy field that animates our mental, emotional, and physical spheres. I believe it emanates from the soul world, and as it goes through each subsequent dimension of the human being, it takes on the nature of that world – so it animates thoughts and beliefs in the dimension of the mind, it takes on the nature of feelings in the emotional dimension, and it condenses itself into a more tangible form in the physical realm. The difference between a person sitting alive one moment, and then being dead the next, simply involves the passing on of the Vital Force animated by the soul outside of the body.

Everything's physical manifestation reflects its inner essence.
Jakob Bohme (1575 – 1624)

Homeopathy taught me something that may have slipped my awareness had I not encountered it in my studies and practice – The idea of symptoms being an expression of the Vital Force's mistunement and what happens when we try to deal with those symptoms in various ways. Let's start by looking at the allopathic way which involves trying to combat the symptoms by suppressing them or in other words, giving some supplement, drug or agent known to remove that symptom or condition from the body. The metaphor I find so helpful to understand in this topic is that of a screaming, crying child. The child is upset, that is clear. The crying and screaming is an expression or symptom of that upset. The allopathic approach, because it involves addressing the symptoms and the source of the upset, would seek some intervention like sticking a sock in the child's throat or putting duct tape over the mouth. This would, in the short run, initially stop the expressing of the upset. But what happens to the upset in this case? Because the outward expression of the upset has been shut down or suppressed, the inner upset, *at its source*, worsens. As it worsens, it gets stronger in its need to outwardly express its inner disturbance or mistunement. So the child will either push so hard internally at the constrains of its expression, or it will create a shunt so that the malcontent can be heard, seen or expressed elsewhere, like with steam shooting out of the ears, or the eyes bulging out, or kicking and scratching, or ripping up the room.

In Holistic Counseling, instead of sticking a sock in the child's mouth, we do the more logical and helpful approach and ask them what's bothering them. Novel idea, isn't it? How many great medical calamities could be avoided by simply investigating with the patient how they are feeling about life and what they are going through. Once they are heard at the very source of their pain and inner turmoil, the source of the symptoms is resolved and there is no further need for the expression of symptoms, which were there only to communicate that something was wrong in the inner world.

Symptoms are therefore the means by which the Vital Force expresses itself. Allowing expression is always more helpful, healing, and restorative than the suppression of the expression. Therefore, a case even without any medical intervention at all where the symptoms are uninhibited in their expression is naturally healthier than a case where a person has gone to see their allopathic practitioner and has been put on some drug or supplement and has successfully wiped out the expression of the symptoms.

We see two phenomena in allopathic medicine that further supports this point. The first is physiological adaptation to a certain dosage of a drug or supplement, and the next is the rebound effect after those allopathic measures are removed. In physiological adaptation to a drug/supplement we see a need to continually increase the dosage of a drug or supplement over time in a given case. Why? Because the Vital Force fights back in order to be able to have its symptom expressed externally against the suppression of the drug or supplement. As it fights back, the inner disturbance in the Vital Force gets stronger, as anything does as it fights an adversary, thus the need for continually higher doses of the drug or supplement at hand.

In the rebound effect, the same phenomenon is occurring as in physiological adaptation. We see a strong burst in the expression of symptoms once the suppressive drug or supplement is removed. Let's take the case of constipation. In constipation, the body is playing the faithful puppy dog of emulating what is going on in the Vital Force of the person in the level of the mind and emotion. As I stated earlier, I have noted constipation involves some form of "holding onto crap/waste" in a person's life. Some toxic, unhealthy emotional baggage that is tagging along that the person won't rid themselves of. The body responds to the "master's" intention (mind) to hold onto crap by obediently doing the same. Along comes the allopathic measure – some form of laxative that tries to push out the faeces whilst at the same time, the mind/Vital Force is giving the command to the body to hold onto the faeces. Imagine the tug of war that ensues, as the Vital Force must push against the adversarial intent of the laxative. At first, the laxative may win and the bowels will empty their contents. But that does not sit well with the disturbance in the Vital Force whose intent is to "hold onto waste." So the Vital Force pushes back, harder now, to hold on and the body responds obediently to express the imbalance. The laxative pushes the body against the wishes of its master. So the body strives to overcome the oppositional element inside of itself. The rebound effect occurs because the force that was pushing against the intent of the Vital Force is suddenly removed; this results in a great lurch forward of the intent of the Vital Force to express its imbalance or mistunement via way of the symptoms. Like when someone is pushing against a door and then the door is suddenly opened, the person lurches forward into the doorway. Thus, understanding the ways of the Vital Force helps us recognize the underlying mechanics of physiological adaptation and the rebound effect in the allopathic approach.

Another travesty occurs when the external suppressive force of the drug or supplement is just too strong for the Vital Force to manage to overcome to any extent at all. Then the pathology must move to a deeper level of the Vital Force in order to express its imbalance. We see this in cases of eczema where the expression of the mistunement is taking place on the level of one of the least vital organs – the skin, and then some suppressive topical drug, like corticosteroid cream, is administered to the eczema. The eczema disappears, but the imbalance moves to a deeper level in the body and hits a more vital organ – the lungs, and the patient develops asthma. Interestingly, when naturopaths and homeopaths have encountered cases of asthma from a history of suppression of eczema, and they work with the Vital Force to clear the asthma, what happens? The eczema returns to the surface of the skin, which reveals another working of the Vital Force. When something is suppressed, it doesn't go away. It just goes deeper into the Vital Force and comes out as a more pathological expression of the Vital Force's mistunement. In fact, having external skin eruptions is a means of the body "dumping out" and expressing its inner disharmony in a most externalizing fashion. To remove this means of externalizing imbalance and toxicity is a sure way to exacerbate a patient's health.

The *Organon* thoroughly discusses this phenomenon and brings many examples of how different diseases can exist in layers at various depths of the Vital Force. Asthma is a more serious and more dangerous form of pathology than eczema on the skin. Samuel Hahnemann, the founder of Homeopathy and author of the *Organon*, made another amazing discovery that relates directly to this subject of suppressing eruptions on the skin, which should be studied and addressed by all healthcare practitioners. Hahnemann discovered that some of his cases were not responding to well-indicated remedies. It perplexed him greatly and he made a point to determine the reason behind the "Law of Similars" not working. He discovered that in those cases that were not responding to the well-indicated remedies, that there was a history or a family history of some form of suppression of the external eruption of certain infectious diseases. He recognized that the suppression of the external eruption of an infectious disease had led to a more serious, more chronic and deeply embedded form of disease in the person that could then be transmitted to offspring. He called this form of chronic disease from the suppression of an external eruption a 'miasm' and he initially dealt with three major miasms – that is, the external suppression of the scabies infection leads to what he called the Psoric miasm. The external suppression of the fig wart in gonorrhoea leads to what he called the Sycotic miasm. And the external suppression of the syphilitic ulcer or bubo in Syphilis, leads to the Syphilitic miasm. These forms of chronic disease are so insidious, so deeply ingrained in the genetic code of the person when they have been passed on through the generations, that they seep into every aspect of a person's life, leaving them a little "less of themselves" just about everywhere across the board.

When I see a miasm in practice, I know I have encountered it because I experience it as the person having been moving along nicely through the questions I am asking them, going deeper and deeper with good progress, only to hit a wall where progress slows down to a crawl and sometimes is stopped entirely. The metaphor I see is like that of a person strolling down a path in the forest, and falling in a pit of quicksand. Hahnemann chose the word "miasm" after the Greek word *miasma* meaning "swamp gas," and it is very much this sort of heavy, insidious, pervasive swamp gas that creeps into a person's mind, emotions and body, casting a darkened cloud over their Vital Force when they have a miasm.

This information is vital to anyone practicing holistically, as most cases are tainted by some form of miasm or another, and often people have more than one miasm. One should be aware of this in order to know what to do – either by addressing the miasm issue with homeopathy, having been trained properly in classical homeopathy, or by referring to a practitioner who has been adequately trained. As subtle and harmless as homeopathy seems, it is nonetheless very potent and requires a lot of study to understand the subtle choices that need to be made in practice. It is not to be dabbled with and contrary to some modern belief, it is possible to harm someone with homeopathy when it is misused or used irresponsibly, without proper education.

I do think it is remotely possible to remove a miasm through Holistic Counseling, although it would take a tremendous amount of skill and experience on the part of the practitioner, and it would require great patience on both the parts of the practitioner and the patient and many sessions. I have made progress in helping people by addressing the fundamental beliefs that reside within their miasms only to see them returned frequently at the next appointments. It is like getting a shovel to dig out a hole in the quicksand. If you dig fast enough, you make an impression, but given a little time, the rest of the quicksand oozes itself back in place and it is as if nothing has happened. One reason for this is that the person has never known anything beside the reality of the miasm, as most are born into this life not knowing any different. With an inherited belief, there is no "healthy" reference in the lifetime experience of the person. Rather, they came in this life subconsciously already carrying some form of block to the Truth and The Healing Power of Nature. It's like the difference between a person who has gone blind earlier in life, versus someone who was born blind. The person who is born blind has no recollection in that life of what anything looks like. It is very hard to draw from a memory that hasn't had the chance to exist. It is said that a cat raised from a kitten in a room that has vertical lines painted on the walls will not be able to see vertical objects that resemble the lines on the wall and will thus bump into things like the legs of a chair or a table. The cat, so "used to" the lines on the wall, stops paying attention to them. This a good metaphor for the subconscious mind of a person who was born into an environment that they have never known to be any different. A person born into a life with the Psoric miasm has never known the peaceful feeling of trusting in the abundance of the Universe. Rather, they live with the constant feeling of insecurity like there is never enough, or as if they are never enough. Holistic Counseling can get a person to this bottom line belief, the source of the struggle inherent in the Psoric miasm, and it may be possible to shake it for some time, and perhaps by repeatedly "challenging" that reality as truth, it could eventually be released. But I see it as so much more challenging than just administering the remedy to neutralize the insidious sticky fog than trying to bat it away with the hands. It's like getting gum on the face. It sticks to the face. If one tries to pull it off, it can smear elsewhere, remain stuck on the face and then spread also onto the hands. In dealing with these miasms homeopathically, we use the very gum that is stuck to remove the gum from the face. The remedy sweeps through and removes the difficult to handle energies by being "like" them – like a chunk of gum picking up more gum unto itself, or like a thicker fog moving through an area of fog, and leaving the air as clear as crystal after it passes through.

If you are working on a case with Holistic Counseling and you notice you keep encountering the same belief in a person and the same thread despite the fact that you know for a fact that the person did have one or more breakthroughs in previous appointments, definitely think about addressing a miasm.

The combination of a practitioner using both Holistic Counseling and homeopathy as a dynamic duo, I believe to be one of the most potent approaches to healing on the planet today. Throw in some form of movement of the body, like Pilates, osteopathy, good massage that gets the whole body moving with the joints, muscles, tendons and ligaments, along with the inner organs, and you're bringing it even further!

The Law of Similars, meaning that like cures like, or using the poison for the cure, that is inherent in homeopathy, is also at the source of all medicines that heal truly in the holistic fashion. To contrast two similar hands-on manipulation techniques – chiropractic and osteopathy – osteopathy from Europe, not the American version which is mostly allopathic and involves little hands-on – osteopathy works with the principle of "like curing like" in a way, by going into the source of the injury until the body unravels itself from the trauma and it is released at its source. Like a ship moored to a dock, the osteopath will bring the ship closer to the dock, facing the source of the problem, in this analogy, being tied up, until there is enough slack to remove the rope gently. The chiropractic approach, rather, is to force the ship out to sea so that the rope essentially breaks. The holistic healer goes into the source of the health issue until it releases so that The Healing Power of Nature can enter and restore health. The allopathic measure, in this case, chiropractic, overpowers the body's tendency to hold on or tighten up against something and forces the body in the opposite direction it is trying to maintain in its expression of disease, or in response to the wound.

Holistic Counseling also works with the "Like cures Like" principle because it helps a person encounter their problem directly at its source. It is not about supplanting some external thought to counterbalance a negative belief. In the *Organon*, Samuel Hahnemann defines psychotherapeutic means as "displays of trust, friendly exhortations, reasoning with the patient, and even well-camouflaged deception."[11] This is exactly the form of psychotherapy that *we do not* employ in the process of Holistic Counseling. For instance, if someone feels they are ugly, we do not say "Oh no, you are so beautiful." Or if someone feels incapable in life, we do not say "Oh, but you are so very capable." That is allopathic counseling – giving something from the outside to counterbalance or oppose the misperception. Rather than doing so, we help a person see their belief as it has been living inside of them. So like cures like, yet instead of a remedy that reflects their pathology, they confront their pathology directly through the uncovering of the hidden beliefs lurking in the subconscious mind. When something is mirrored in this fashion, healing results.

I have just called this allopathic counseling, because it is supplying awareness, either through reason, trust, or encouragement, via the doctor. It becomes a form of a prescription *from the outside*. It therefore does not arise from the wisdom of Nature, or from the patient's own awareness. That is why it does not work to heal or help in any way the deeper forms of illness that have become embedded in the body. Recall that disease is as a result of straying from one's I AM. And the I AM is really only known to the individual, to the person themselves. The doctor cannot really supply that.

So, this form of psychotherapy is specifically to be avoided in the Vis Dialogue process. Hahnemann mentions using this form of psychotherapeutic means to improve a patient's condition under two circumstances. In the first situation he states:

If the mental disease is not yet fully developed and if there is still some doubt as to whether it arose from somatic suffering or whether it stemmed from faulty upbringing, bad habits, perverted morality, neglect of the spirit, superstitions or ignorance, the way to decide the point is as follows:

1. If it stems from the latter [faulty upbringing, bad habits, etc.], then the mental disease will subside and improve with

understanding, well-intentioned exhortations, consolation, or with earnest and rational expostulations.

2. If it is a mental or emotional disease that is really based upon a somatic disease, it will rapidly worsen with such treatment.[11]

And in the second situation where he states that such psychotherapeutic means (that we don't use in Holistic Counseling) will help a condition, he writes:

It is only these emotional diseases, which were first spun and maintained by the soul, that allow themselves to be rapidly transformed into well-being of the soul by psychotherapeutic means (displays of trust, friendly exhortations, reasoning with the patient, and even well-camouflaged deception). With appropriate living habits, these diseases apparently also allow themselves to be transformed into well-being of the body. However, such approaches will be effective *only if the emotional disease is new and has not yet deranged the somatic state all too much*.[11]

So what we know from understanding this section of the *Organon*, and in particular these two aphorisms 224 & 226, is that allopathic psychotherapy can be used to help patients whose mental disease arises from faulty upbringing, bad habits, perverted morality, etc. and also, in emotional diseases, which were first spun and maintained by the soul. We can also interpret from Hahnemann's writing here that an emotional disease spun and maintained by the soul, *given enough time*, will become a somatic disease that affects the body. Once it is at the somatic level, (driven into the body) such allopathic psychotherapeutic means become ineffective and can even worsen the condition. We also know from Hahnemann that allopathic psychotherapeutic means do not help mental or emotional diseases that are also rooted in the body, aka somatic, as it is stated in Aphorism 224 point number 2.

During Hahnemann's time, it is unlikely that there were many forms of counseling or psychotherapy that functioned in a fashion to get to the root cause of illness and release it. So the idea of using counseling or psychotherapy to address disease that had become manifest in the body and thus inherently somatic, was out of the question. Therefore Hahnemann relied entirely upon the homeopathic remedies to employ the use of the Law of Similars. This was truly an effective means of healing, compared to the allopathic world of medicine at the time, and seen today, which is not only ineffective for combatting chronic somatic disease, but also rather harmful and excessive. However, what I have regularly seen happen in my cases using Holistic Counseling, even of physical, somatic diseases, is that, by going deeply into the subconscious mind of the patient, a root cause is arrived at, that is the original choice that led a patient to stray from their true nature. Through the chronicity of time, the subsequent effects of that "false" choice in the mental-emotional sphere brings on a change at the level of the body, as I described in the earlier sections, and the disease does indeed become somatic. It is true that the deeper a disharmony becomes rooted in the body, i.e. somatic, the more embedded it is, and the more difficult it is for it to become released. Hahnemann stated that these somatic diseases can only be cured with the Law of Similars, i.e. with homeopathic remedies that fit the totality of the strange, rare, and peculiar symptoms, matching the somatic symptoms, as well as the mental-emotional state (Aphorisms 213, 214, 220). What I would like to add now to this understanding is that it does not mean that employing the Law of Similars through counseling to help a patient "see" what is their problem, is not akin to the Law of Similars. We can say this in another way. By helping to reveal the root cause of the disease and helping the patient release the underlying choice that led to their illness, these somatic illnesses can be cured. In some cases, it takes longer than at other times to bring about the healing on all levels. But it can and it does happen. The bottom line is that Hahnemann's take on psychotherapy or counseling during his time is nothing like what is accomplished in Holistic Counseling as I am offering it today. And even physical disease can be cured using nothing more than non-directional questions to reveal the root cause of a patient's problem to them.

There are, however, some situations where the disease is simply too far embedded and cannot be arrived at without the help of homeopathy and other modalities that work in harmony with the Vis to release the illness from all levels of the being. This is discussed in Chapter 36 on the *Limitations of Holistic Counseling* towards the end of the book.

The next important function we fulfill in Holistic Counseling is to help the patient then see that it is in fact a choice that they are believing something harmful, distorted, or misaligned with their true nature, and not a carved-in-stone absolute reality, even if their problem has become manifest somatically. In Part III on the Vis Dialogue of Holistic Counseling, I will explain how to go about that with the use of certain questions strategically timed and other techniques to use to reveal the underlying choice and how to let it go. Homeopathy also fulfills this same function of revealing the underlying belief that led to an illness, yet more subtly and at times, solely through the wisdom of Nature speaking. Sometimes, following a good remedy, and the clarity that comes from the old, blocked energies being cleared, the choices a person has been making that have been unhealthy for them rise to the surface of the conscious mind and no longer seem like a viable option any longer. It is amazing to watch Nature teach a patient through this process. Other times, however, the awareness may not even reach a person's conscious mind when they begin to choose a healthier way to live. Changes can take place deeply in the realm of dreams, or in the shadowy places of the subconscious mind, so very subtly and slowly allowing for change that a person never becomes conscious of the actual choice they made to be healthier and more aligned with their true nature. This is also amusing to observe in practice because patients may even be under the impression that the remedy didn't do anything. I cannot count how many times it has happened in practice where I have asked my patients, "*So how was it taking the remedy?*" Answer, "I didn't feel much. It didn't do anything." And then I will ask, "*How are the headaches?*" Answer, "What headaches?" or, "*How is the anxiety?*" Answer, "What anxiety?" So subtly did the remedy heal them that they didn't even remember that their chief complaint was headaches or anxiety. One of the things I love about the combination of using Holistic Counseling and homeopathy together is that the underlying core belief is brought to light from the dark recesses of the subconscious mind and then the homeopathic remedy hits it right between the eyes. It's like that old arcade game where a person would use a big bat to hit gophers on the head as they came up out of holes in the machine. This combination really facilitates a patient's change of mind.

It should be noted that even though I love the combo of these two phenomenal holistic forms of healing, it is my very favorite form of healing to help a person heal even the toughest of physical diseases, strictly by helping them recognize the unhealthy choice about their reality that led to their illness and then choosing to let it go through Holistic Counseling. It is, as Dr. Paul Epstein calls, "homeopathy without the remedy." I find this is the most empowering form of healing for a patient. It is the form of healing that is simplest, the most cost-effective, and enabling *doctor as teacher* to be empowered in the most profound way, because the practitioner is helping a person see how their illness was engendered via their negative belief. This reveals to the patient their true Nature and brings them closer to the

Creator with nothing but the use of reflective questions. When I see a person has really gotten to the core of their illness and has chosen to let that false choice go, I will refrain from giving any other recommendations so as to not interfere with this most pure and valuable experience. It's only when I see them struggling with the core, or they return and there has not been much progress that I will employ the use of homeopathy to assist in the process.

Chapter 10

What is the Subconscious Mind?

The subconscious mind seems to be a great realm of mystery. Because it is so shrouded and beyond the understanding of the conscious mind, we have so often classified it as beyond reach. I have found, however, that through Holistic Counseling, given enough time and enough well-placed questions, a person can contact levels of their subconscious that were previously far beyond their awareness. Even in only one session, I have seen people go from being in complete darkness regarding the forces that govern them from their subconscious, to becoming completely aware of the thread and the theme of the limiting belief system that runs through their lives that has dictated their behavior, influenced their health and restricted their view of reality.

So what is the subconscious mind, really? I believe the subconscious mind is the part of the conscious mind that used to be conscious, but became buried under layers of repetitive thoughts and habits such that one forgot what one was actually thinking. Like the way in which the brain has the ability to "tune out" something that is going on constantly, like the buzz of a light bulb in the ceiling, or the sound of traffic from a distant highway, so too can the mind "tune out" the repetitive thoughts which underlie our reality. Things go into the "back of the mind." That is another good way of understanding the subconscious mind. The subconscious and conscious minds are therefore connected along one seamless and continual thread. At one time, a thought was in the conscious mind until one may have thought it so often, for so long and so continually and chronically, that one simply stopped consciously paying attention to it. It then slipped into the realm of the subconscious.

The oldest thoughts that went into the subconscious are the most deeply buried, because as new conscious thoughts became so repeated, they were consciously ignored and also slipped into the subconscious, burying the deeper layers of the subconscious that much more. We are born with thoughts buried in the subconscious mind that we inherited from our ancestors (genetic and miasmatic), that come from past lives, and that also come from the collective consciousness of the human "condition."

The oldest buried thoughts in the subconscious are also the most influential. They are the oldest and the deepest forms of limiting beliefs that influence the flow of The Healing Power of Nature and alter our Vital Force. Like a house of cards, the oldest layers in the subconscious act as a foundation for the rest of the layers of the subconscious built up on them. For example, a child is abandoned when very young and begins to think and feel that the world is not a safe place. The child holds onto this thought as a means of justifying the pain of their abandonment. They think it long enough that it becomes a "no-brainer" – a belief that has been thought for so long that it slips effortlessly into the quiet darkness of the subconscious mind. Since the world is believed to be an unsafe place, this layer will lead the child to never quite feel at ease. This subconscious layer will then act as a foundation for other similar beliefs to "build up" further layers. Later the child, then older, may experience their first heartbreak in romance. Following this trauma, they begin to think "love relationships are not safe." This they may think long enough, state to themselves and others enough that this next layer becomes integrated into their subconscious and is the next deepest layer to the belief that life, itself, is not safe. Further traumas in life could then conglomerate with these initial, deepest layers and lead to other beliefs and thoughts, held on by the wounded person, such as "men are not to be trusted (unsafe)," "friends are not to be trusted (unsafe)" etc. Since life is unsafe, one can then believe they must do everything alone. There is no one there to help. Then, since everything must be done alone, the next belief stacked onto the house of cards could constitute that everything is such effort. I cannot make it in this world. Life is too hard. Later, due to this disconnect, even seemingly unrelated beliefs can take hold on the upper levels of the stack of cards. The possibilities of the combination of different beliefs are really, endless, and it is why we must work with each person as an individual, because each case is made up of such very unique beliefs and patterns of wounding.

In a case with a woman with body dysmorphic disorder (issues with her body's appearance), we began working with her relationship with herself and how it played out in her life. When we explored the issue, it came down to feeling not important, not good enough. This feeling, when we explored it, was brought up by her parents fighting and her being in the middle. She felt like she was just there to convey messages of how her parents hated each other, but she, in essence, meant nothing to her parents. Thus was developed this feeling of being unimportant and the subsequent need to compensate by comparing herself to others and needing to look a certain way. In recognizing this and making changes around her perception of herself, she began to feel much better and was really improving.

Then we had a follow-up and she consulted me for some other present issues. The follow-up really depicts how these layers can appear, and how, like a house of cards, one issue stands upon the layer of another. She had two things she wanted to discuss with me. One was, "I get into this place where I don't know what to do with myself. It's not exactly a boredom, but like, an inability to find what I want to do, what excites me or makes me happy."

The second issue was that she was comparing herself again to others, but not in terms of her body's appearance. It was more like in terms of how much a person had their "shit together."

Upon exploring via the Holistic Counseling questions, it

became clear that she felt really good when she felt needed. In places where people needed her advice and her help, she felt great. But when she was around people who didn't need her, and were possibly even (in her perception) "a bigger light than her," she would feel unneeded, not worthy of anybody's attention, and like "Ehhh, not important." She also felt like she needed to be the best, biggest, brightest light, and most expert in a given niche. At this point, she realized that the first issue she had brought up during this particular follow-up, of not knowing what to do with herself, was related to this. She recognized that she felt she didn't know what to do with herself because she felt the need to do something great, something big, the best, amazing thing, and if she didn't, there was no point in doing anything. So, these two issues that she wanted to deal with converged into one. Upon further investigation, she was able to make the connection that this came from the need to feel needed and important and worthy of people's attention. I asked her what the opposite of that was? (This is an advanced question in the Vis Dialogue.) She said, "Unneeded, unworthy of people's time, and unimportant." So then I asked her if there was anywhere else in her life where she felt this same way? (This is called a "Reflecting-Elsewhere" question.) And she said, yes, with her father and her mother. Upon exploration, it was revealed that her mother left her when she was a very young child. From this, she had concluded that she was unneeded, unimportant and not worthy of her mother's time, which then got translated in her mind as not just for her mother, but globally. That was the original wound and her deepest core belief – being unneeded, unworthy of people's time, and unwanted. This was the base of the house of cards. The body dysmorphic disorder was the first, and uppermost layer we worked on, but what helped initially, was dealing with the base of the house of cards, which in this particular follow-up, was revealed in the most deep and the most "root-cause" fashion. She then sought to counterbalance this core belief and feeling by compensating to be the best, and brightest in a given niche so that she could feel others needed her, she was worthy of their time, and she felt wanted by them. This compensation could be seen on the layer of her house of cards where she had an issue of not feeling like doing anything. A lethargy, lack of motivation, all because she felt she needed to be the best and the most amazing before she did anything at all, which is impossible to fulfill, hence the inactivity and lethargy. It could also be seen on another level of the house of cards with her father, whom she felt didn't care about her. When we explored it, he didn't seem interested in having a close relationship with her. This made her feel yet again... unimportant. She recognized that all these different issues she was carrying around on different levels of the house of cards, all sat upon the foundation that was initially started with the wound of her mother. The house of cards, therefore, could begin coming down. And so it did and with it, the issues that had been causing her a lot of suffering. The first complaint, body dysmorphic disorder, was also related to the lower level of the house of cards as she needed her body to look a certain way to get attention as a means of compensating for not feeling important.

In another case of a woman, we had several appointments and continued to get deeper and deeper toward the root of her problems. She said, "It scares me – I feel I am finally getting to the inside layers and it is just getting harder. Not easier." Healing, at times, unfolds slowly. Each step of healing of a layer and going deeper provides the tools, the courage, the experience, the trust, and the confidence to deal with the next deepest layer. Eventually, when a person faces their greatest challenge, i.e. that which lives at the deepest buried level of their Vital Force and their subconscious, it will feel the most challenging for them, and involves the greatest healing. For some cases, the patient cannot have arrived right to the bottom layer in the first session or first few sessions. It's simply too suppressed, too painful. It requires a step-wise fashion, growing with each step, readying for further healing. The practitioner must remember this and not expect every case to resolve during the first few appointments. We didn't get our patients sick and we are not responsible, per se, of getting them better. Our responsibility is to show up and help them heal as expediently as possible, but how quickly that occurs is determined by the severity, depth, and nature of the wounds that the patient carries. And yes, a practitioner, in time, with more experience, will be able to help cases in a more expedient fashion by knowing how to help get a patient to the core quicker and with less fuss.

One can only deal with the most recent trauma-turned-belief at a time, but that is not to say that one cannot cycle down through more than one layer of the subconscious in a given session of Holistic Counseling. In some cases, it is just not possible to do more than one layer at a time, as the magnitude of the force of emotion that accompanies each layer is just too powerful and influential and the pain too suppressed and resisted for too long to get through more than a little at a time. However, depending on the practitioner and the patient, it is possible to get to the very bottom layer in one session. It really astounds me when I see how much a person can come in touch with that they had "forgotten" or buried. The subconscious mind to the Holistic Counseling practitioner is not so out of reach and mysterious. We can prove this through the simple action of asking a string of questions designed to get the person thinking deeper and deeper into the workings of their mind.

Part II

Principles and Metaphors for a Wholesome Holistic Practice

The following are wholesome principles that I have observed while working with people. It has served me very well in practicing Holistic Counseling. Normally, the practitioner does not teach or talk during practice. I know how frustrating it can be to be with a counselor or psychotherapist who teaches and talks a lot. After seeing how effective Holistic Counseling is, I know that this form of therapy with the therapist doing a lot of the talking is not very effective. In Holistic Counseling, we don't do that. We simply ask questions. So, these following metaphors are mostly for the understanding of the practitioner, but they can be used where the opportunity calls for it and seems appropriate. There are certain key times, when a person hesitates out of the sheer novelty of what they are undergoing, or you can tell they are resisting from inside their own perception of reality, and it can be of great benefit to share a brief outline of one or more of the following principles and metaphors. And it is not like we are giving a lecture about their core and most deep belief system, trying to convince them it is untrue. These principles and metaphors are helpful at a specific time when the dialogue itself is being affected by a person's perception of their healing, of counseling, of confusing one thing for another. I will also use metaphors to loosen the tension around very locked in beliefs that are stuck and not responding well to the questions. I've found cases that were not advancing well open right up after I shared 'The Two Paths' or the 'Error in Innocence' and other metaphors. I do this briefly, concisely, so we can move onto more open-ended, non-directional questions. If I find myself using too many metaphors, I know I am being too controlling in the Holistic Counseling.

Chapter 11

The Two Paths and the Compensation

This is the metaphoric principle I share the most with patients during practice. I find that after sharing it, they will begin to understand themselves better and know which path they are walking on. The Two Paths metaphor is very profound and can shed light on the direction a person has been following their entire life. Students and practitioners also find it very helpful to reflect on their own "Physician, Heal Thyself!" path.

Basically, in life, there is, in essence, one of two paths we can follow. The first is the path of Truth. It is our true nature, our calling, our heart's truest wishes, and the fulfillment of our purpose. It is the path we follow in being our true selves. It is essentially walk our I AM statement. Our soul's being. It is healthy. It is empowering. It is living on the cutting edge of life. It is, however, not without challenge. In fact, it is likely on this path that we encounter the most challenges, because the world tends to throw up many obstacles for a person to overcome in order to be their true selves. And on this path, it is necessary for a person to face their fears. We can say that fears stand in the way of us being ourselves. Once we have stepped into the center of our core, that is, the heart of our true nature, there is no more fear. But to get there requires facing fears because so long as we are not being ourselves totally and completely, then there will be some fear standing in the way of us returning to the essence of our being. So, the first path of Truth requires the facing of fears.

The second of the two paths is the exact opposite. It is a path where we run from our fears. A fear can seem so very frightening, overwhelming, and undesirable, that a person can literally run away from their fear their entire lives. The desire to *not* experience their fear can become such a strong pull that the person begins to truly believe that what they want is the second path, to not have their fear happen, and so whatever way they have chosen to run away from their fear seems like what they truly want. We can also say that a person on the second path chooses equally to run from their wound. The wound, therefore, becomes a fear, and they choose to run from it.

This second path is based on an illusion. It is a path of nothingness.

For example, Little Timmy is playing in a sandbox with some friends. Timmy is a little chubby. The other children are mean and make fun of him and then leave him to play by himself in the sandpit. The wound strikes Timmy so deeply and is so painful that he makes a strong statement to himself, "I will never let anyone ever make fun of me again." So Timmy works hard to avoid any situation, and every situation, where he could be made fun of, initially perhaps regarding his weight or his physique, but then later extending into intellectual achievement in school, and physical performance in sports. He works out, intent on getting rid of the weight. He combs his hair perfectly so others will find it attractive. He speaks carefully, so that nothing he says seems silly and can be laughed at.

One can say that within the second path are certainly some ways of being that are desirable to anyone. Exercise. Good hygiene. Studying hard during school. Yet it is the underlying intention behind a behavior that matters more than the act itself. So exercising is great. Exercising to look good to avoid being ridiculed is not good for a person's life. It is always in relationship to the wound and *therefore continually feeds the wound*. The second path, therefore, always maintains the fear intact and the more activity we do to avoid the fear, the stronger the fear gets. The second path, therefore, always leads to some form of illness or dis-ease. Initially, the dis-ease lives in the mental emotional sphere and later, in the body.

What also happens on the second path is that a person grows

up and they don't even know what they really want or who they really are. Timmy spends so much time avoiding the fear of being ridiculed that he lives as a shadow of himself, making choices always out of running from fear, rather than what he really wants. Holistic Counseling will always bring this schism to the surface. If Timmy were in my office, I would likely have to explain this metaphor to him, otherwise, while counseling him and asking him the question *"Do you want to keep living this way?"* he might not understand that what he really wants is to stop running from his fear. What he really wants is not all the ego-boosting success or praise, but rather to just be at peace being himself, unafraid of what others think of him. That is true success. That is true freedom and the first of the two paths will bring that to someone that pursues it. In this way, we can see that Holistic Counseling does bring a person to confront Truth and make choices to align with it.

The first path of being true to self involves facing one's fear, and is healthy, fortifying. The second path brings a person further and further away from their true nature. It is the path that leads to illness. So we can see that running from fear causes illness. It is akin to the way in which suppressing disease causes more disease.

I see many people with a core underlying fear of being abandoned. Ultimately, we could even see that in Timmy, who fears being ridiculed because then people don't like him and he will be left alone to play by himself. We are social creatures, and nurture ourselves largely from the love we receive from others. People who have the fear of being abandoned often get into the unbalanced feminine energy, where they do things for others so that others will like them and not want to leave them. Doing for others is nice. Doing for others so that others will like you so that they don't abandon you is a false front and lies on the second of two paths.

I have noticed that people often get sick when the youthful

energy to flee from their fears runs out. The amount of energy a person has to run from their fears is always finite. There is always a breaking point where their life simply cannot sustain it. It is at this point that disease can really manifest and that they begin to seek healing. In their youth, they have plenty of energy to build up the life of "not" – not poor, not ridiculed, not alone, not stupid, not left out, not not-good enough – but as they age, this energy ebbs and eventually dries up, and they are left simply not able to run anymore. They cannot continue creating a life with a false foundation, nor can they continue to run from their fears. In fact, I believe the illness comes on for this very purpose – to reveal to the person the emptiness of the second path. And it should be so, because running from fear is the exact opposite direction from where a person truly wants to be. In their heart of hearts, and in the higher self that guides them, through fear and toward our true self is the direction we all wish to travel. Herein lies another aspect of the mystery of The Healing Power of Nature. It is aligned with Truth. It calls us back to know our true selves, even if we are consciously still desirous of goals that are not healthy for us. It does so by helping to manifest illness so that we can learn. That is a truly novel way of looking at disease, in contrast with the combative, totally insensitive forms of allopathic and conventional medicine.

The Compensation on the Second Path

Whenever we walk on the second path of running from our fears, we choose a behavior or a way of thinking to counterbalance the fear. This an attempt to compensate for the fear. Timmy worked extra hard on his physical appearance, on his social skills, on his grades, on the job he had, all in order to compensate for the fear of being ridiculed. A person who does everything for everyone else to be loved by them so they won't be abandoned is using the "doing for everyone" behavior as a compensation for their fear of being abandoned. The compensation is always counterbalancing the fear so it is always staying in relationship to it. It never goes away. It just gets stronger by trying to compensate and counter-balance it. In fact, the compensation behavior cannot exist without the underlying fear. Explaining this to a person can change their life on the spot. They will see how their behavior is actually stemming out of the fear of their fear and not based in who they are or what they truly want.

I had a case of a young woman who had a hard time loving herself. She felt unable to fulfill her potential, she struggled with feeling attractive, and it was very difficult for her to love herself. Her compensation was to help others see how very beautiful they were and how much potential they had which they were not fulfilling. It gave her such a great joy that she revolved her entire life around trying to make this possible. The trouble is, the more she did so, she would only have brief glimpses of feeling good about herself, but the wound and lack of love for herself lived on. And because the wound and lack of love lived on, she had to make that much more effort to help others, which was depleting her and led to her become exhausted and unhappy.

A person who aims to please everyone to be liked so as to not be abandoned, eventually loses their ability to continue to do so. From lack of nurturing themselves, they simply run out of steam and are no longer capable of running around, pleasing everyone. Timmy could eventually develop a stomach ulcer from drinking too much coffee in order to keep him going on his path of impressing people and also from all the stress in his third chakra relating to his feelings of low self-esteem. With the ulcer, he would have to stop drinking coffee, which would slow him down and make it hard for him to go to the gym, or to work as many extra hours as he does. At his slower, less impressive pace, he will be forced to face his fears. With more serious pathology, he will be forced to face his fear even more intensely.

When a person runs out of energy to compensate for their wound, they cannot do the compensating behavior any longer.

What results is that their fear surfaces. This is Nature's way and the Creator's way of making us face our fears so we can learn to love ourselves and be true to ourselves. They may express their chief complaint as an inability or a lack of energy to do what they want to do. But it's really the energy running out to continue on the second of the two paths. Really, it is as a result of something deeper which must be faced and the Holistic practitioner can really help them see that and help them change their entire life. Imagine what is happening when allopathic practitioners are just boosting up the person's adrenals and supporting them with other adaptogenic herbs and supplements so they can keep chasing an empty path, running from their fears?

The compensation is like a drug. To "accomplish" it brings one a feeling of happiness, success, accomplishment. The woman who made others feel good about themselves felt so good when she could help someone. She felt soft and blissful inside. But it was short lived. The poor relationship with herself continued and the wound needed to be fed from the outside to make her feel good about herself again. Timmy needs success to make himself feel better, as the compensation monster in him gets hungry. And as he feeds the beast of the compensation, like with physiological adaption from any drug, the underlying wound gets stronger, pushing back against the outer 'drug,' and so Timmy needs to feed the beast more and more. Being a manager is not enough. He needs to be upper management, then he needs to be CEO.

This is such a helpful metaphor. When sharing it to help someone who is stuck believing they actually desire what they are using to compensate and to run from their fear, it is important to explain the part about the compensation.

Chapter 12

Error in Innocence

When a child adopts a belief that is not in harmony with their true nature and with Creation, they are making an error in innocence. They don't know any better. They don't know that their father not being around very much is not a negative reflection of themselves. The absence of the father hurts, and the child concludes it must be something wrong with them. The fact that they don't know any better is based in their innocence. But the fact nevertheless remains that they chose a reality which is simply incorrect in the big picture of things. It is an error. A child who grows up watching his/her family always stuffing their emotions down and keeping a "stiff upper lip" is most definitely innocent of their error when they begin to emulate their parents. The choice doesn't appear to be a choice to the child, because the parents are the most influential examples to be emulated. And yet each day, each year that passes, that same error is perpetuated when the child grows up and becomes an adult, continuing to stuff down their own emotions.

That child grows into an adult, but the inner child lives ever on, frozen in age at the time when the emotions became stuck and unable to grow. Children have vivid imaginations, able to fabricate stories of wild imaginings. These same imaginations spin ideas about the nature of reality that become the core beliefs that imprison the inner child and the grown adult to that limited perspective of reality. The vivid imagination of the inner children I observe often conclude, "I am not lovable because..." and "I am not good enough because" of some major or minor occurrence that is happening in their childhood environment. But the vivid imagination can take on much more creative and flamboyant expressions which can result in a perpetuated error in innocence.

Does the innocent error ever turn not innocent? It doesn't ever, really, because its basis is in innocence, and so, the error is always based in the same spaces where it was spawned. Even subsequent layers of the house of cards are also of an innocent kind, because they are built upon the original error in innocence. However, once one becomes aware of the error, as through Holistic Counseling, then the error must be corrected and the choice must be made to live a fuller and happier life. To wilfully continue to make the same limiting choice following full awareness of its problematic nature is to delve into the realm of the non-innocent. This is not to say that we cannot stumble and wrestle with our limiting beliefs once we've recognized them as such. It can take time to work through old belief systems. And it doesn't mean it is evil or a cardinal sin to continue to live a belief even after it has been recognized. However, as one continues to live the same error, each subsequent time one returns will have more and more serious consequences (this is discussed further in Chapter 18 *"Intolerance of Time and Repetition,"* a few chapters ahead).

This principle is a nice balance of male and female. The unbalanced female energy cringes at such a harsh word as 'error' and would rather make up some nice story to justify the ok-ness of the person's choice. To recognize error is to be empowered to make a change. This is where the male in us thrives. The female works well with the understanding that it was in an innocent state that the diversion from one's true nature came to be. Things that are balanced between male and female, like the concept of *Error in Innocence*, tend to be more effective than unbalanced principles. If we just told someone, "Your belief is an error," it is harsh and lacking grace and compassion. If we just tell people, whatever you believe is ok, or you're still the innocent child you have always been, we lack the discernment to pick ourselves up and choose a healthier and better life for ourselves.

Chapter 13

The Universality of the Truth vs Individualized Perception of Reality

There has been a lot of control surrounding the Truth. People have died for their beliefs, and others have killed for theirs. As a result of this shady past, many in our modern, "New Age" times have adopted an attitude that essentially states, "Whatever anyone believes is the Truth." Even though this is a much more peaceful, flexible and harmonious relationship with Truth, it is still not balanced. No one can ever force the Truth on anyone, and we must all choose the Truth for ourselves. Sometimes the path is long and filled with "missteps" in order to gain clarity around some aspects of the Truth. And even if one were so blessed to have experience of the Truth and knew it, to convey that Truth from one to another is not possible through rational language. As a horse is led to water, one can be led toward the pool of Truth, but to drink is always the choice of the individual, and not of the "guide."

The old way of imposing Truth, killing for Truth, and controlling for Truth is an unbalanced form of the male energy. The idea that whatever anyone believes is the Truth, is a form of the unbalanced female energy. Yes, we can say that what a person believes as Truth has the appearance and experience for them of being true. That does not make it universally true. Believing something to be true, for example, "sex is bad," can bring about a self-fulfilling prophecy. When there is a negative judgment around something like our sexuality from an inherent belief, the mind, as we shared in the section on chakras and Holism, will affect the flow of the chakras so that the belief imposes itself on reality. The "bad" idea on the second/sexual chakra blocks it from flowing naturally and nourishing the body in a healthy fashion.

What results is a blocked 2nd chakra which feels, in simple terms, bad. Any stirring of sexual energy or experience will feel blocked, which feels bad, which is a confirmation of the belief. Any attempt to have sexual relations, living under the canopy of the belief, will not have a free and healthy experience, and will equally confirm the belief. In addition to that, people tend to focus toward what resonates with what they believe. Rape, pornography, sexually transmitted diseases could all be the focus of someone believing sex is bad, rather than the beautiful, healing, ecstatic nature of love making. So, yes, it is true to say that what one believes will have the appearance of Truth in this world. It does not mean that what one believes is the capitol T Truth. The capitol T Truth is that sexuality can be a divine realm to experience pleasure, love, and communion with another. There are many sacred practices of sexuality in some of the ancient traditions of the world, like Kama Sutra in the ancient Vedic Hindu culture. There is Chinese sacred sexuality. Alchemy has a tradition of the sacredness of the sexual union and these teachings also exist in Kabbalah. In short, sexuality can be experienced in myriad ways, and there is always something of the sacred and the divine in it. That is why it has been such a target for control and perversion, because that is the nature of the world – to target and attempt to pervert that which is most sacred. That is why to believe that sex is bad, is understandable, but it is wrong in regards to the Universality of the Truth.

So, why am I sharing all of this? Because in Holistic Counseling, it is important for the practitioner to have a compass on the subject of the Universality of Truth. This is not to say that one sits there and dictates to the patient what is true from what is not, or that one takes the high horse seat and teaches the patient the Truth. That would be a most crude error in Holistic Counseling. Rather, it is important to continue to guide a patient until they arrive at the Universal Truth inside of themselves, and to continue to ask the questions until they get there. That is the balance between the male and the female – the patient must arrive at the Truth for themselves. When one arrives at the Universal Truth, there is healing, there is resonance, and there is peace. They are plugged back into the source of life and The Healing Power of Nature can restore its flow. God flows through The Healing Power of Nature and since God is also Truth, then the Truth and The Healing Power of Nature are also one and the same. Any belief that is not universally true is a block to the experience of Nature's healing power. It's as simple as that. Of course, one's experience of the Universal Truth and one's expression of it will differ from others, as each of us is an individual. But in essence, we can all understand one another.

It is important to recognize that we do not have a grasp on the full picture of the Truth. It is helpful to be aware of certain Universal Truths while practicing Holism, however, it is not an absolute must, otherwise, Holistic Counseling would be based on the knowledge of the practitioner and not on The Healing Power of Nature emanating from the I AM inside the patient. A practitioner can get into unchartered territories for themselves regarding the Truth and still, by asking the patient the next open-ended question to get them to go deeper, can still greatly help them. (And learn something in the process.)

When cases of disease revolve around beliefs that are of a strong religious nature, it is very difficult to do Holistic Counseling to resolve the conflict, because the belief is so locked in, so very certain in the person's mind, and there are large consequences, including social, religious, and spiritual, for letting go of some beliefs. It is for this reason that I have found religious beliefs to be one of the limitations of Holistic Counseling, where the religious belief itself is underlying the person's diseased state. It is a very touchy subject and a practitioner cannot really teach or tell the religious person that their beliefs are in error and/or limiting them or causing them to be sick. One can ask, however, by arriving at the religious belief system through Holistic

Counseling, *"Do you want to keep living this way?"* Who knows? Maybe they have been pondering their own liberation from the extreme religious sect or pathway they are on. The Healing Power of Nature is ever hovering around our minds, waiting to penetrate beyond our limited thinking. So, one should not establish any immediate stance against someone who is religious, thinking, they cannot be helped with Holistic Counseling, because anything is possible. More and more people seem to be leaving the fold of their religious orthodox organizations, just as the world is healing in regards to very controlled religious thought. I published an article about a woman who was sick with myasthenia gravis due to her religious beliefs and life situation. I was able to help her be symptom free with the combination of Holistic Counseling and homeopathy, but it took quite a long time to loosen the bonds to those strong beliefs.[12]

As a balance: There is also another phenomenon happening quite a lot these days, where people are throwing out God with the dirty religious bathwater, along with many of the beautiful Universal Truths that are taught in religion. This, in my opinion, is not in balance and is a sign of lack of discernment, to be unable to separate the good from the bad.

Chapter 14

When Natural, Healthy Responses are Mingled with an Added Unhealthy-Element

Parents wish to keep their children safe. That is natural and healthy. But when they live in constant fear of their children being unsafe, that is having an added unhealthy element mingled into the equation. A woman can have a strong desire to bear children. That is natural and healthy. But if a woman needs to have children to such a degree that her very being depends on it, that has an additional unhealthy element mingled into the equation. A person wishes to get a well-paying job. Natural and healthy. When a person needs to have a well-paying job in order to be happy, or because their reputation or ego depends on it that has an unhealthy element mingled into the natural and healthy.

In some cases, it may be important to just illustrate this concept for a person who believes they want something and their desire is entirely healthy or natural. I had a case of a man in his thirties who had a son and two daughters. After a hospitalization of one of his daughters, he began to become obsessively fearful for both of his daughters' well-being. As we began going deeper into his fear with Holistic Counseling, I could tell he was becoming increasingly uncomfortable with where the questions were leading him. He felt he was being "asked" (through the process of questions) to let go of something that was, for him, healthy and very fundamentally natural. I then realized I should simply provide him with this most simple distinction. "Of course, your desire as a father to keep your children safe and healthy is a very normal, natural, and healthy instinct. But do you think that it is also healthy, normal, and natural to be so very afraid about their health every day in the way that you do?" He thought for a moment and said, "No." So then I said, "So where there is a natural desire, there can also be an unhealthy desire intermingled. What we're doing now is exploring to see what is behind the unhealthy desire so that you can continue to have a natural and healthy instinct as a father to protect and provide for your children, while being at peace and not being kept up at night being so worried about it."

We then continued to explore his life and beliefs that had resulted in him developing myasthenia gravis. Through the Vis Dialogue, what was uncovered was that he first had developed symptoms when he realized the degree to which his younger sister, mostly, and his younger brother, had become serious alcoholics. He had always felt a strong desire to protect his younger siblings from his mother's alcoholism and her terrible, abusive moods. When he couldn't stand being at home with his mother any longer, he left, and had left his two younger siblings, which he described as what felt like, being at the mercy of their mother. He felt guilty for that but knew he had to leave. Years later, when he discovered how much his sister was struggling in her life, he felt responsible and that he had failed to protect her. With this came guilt and the beginning of myasthenia gravis. It was then, during this same period of time, that he began to develop the fear of something happening to his daughters. Interestingly enough, as he came to realize, he wasn't worried about his son. He felt his son was robust enough that he didn't need so much protection. His son, in his mind, did not remind him or resonate with his two younger siblings that he believed he had failed to protect and that he was responsible for their downfall into alcoholism. His daughters, seeming to him frail and more vulnerable, did remind him of his other two "helpless" siblings, especially after one of his daughters was hospitalized from a bad flu that led to breathing problems. So as a father, his instinct to protect, which was healthy and normal, had an added element of great fear and guilt relating to his own siblings which he was attempting to redeem inside of himself by not allowing anything to happen to his daughters (control & compensation). By uncovering this root and these belief systems, and helping him to distinguish between the healthy and unhealthy aspects of being a father, not only did his great fear towards his children dissipate, but his symptoms of myasthenia gravis also improved. They were all related.

Another case example on this topic is of a woman who wanted to have children. That is a natural and healthy inclination. Her husband wasn't sure and was taking a lot of time deciding whether or not he wanted to have children. She then began to put pressure and stated that if he didn't want to have children, she would leave the relationship and then seek out another partner who could fulfill her wishes. So far, this is all normal and natural and balanced, healthy responses. The trouble was that the woman also had an accompanying unhealthy element mingled with her natural desire. The background of the story is that she had a very hard life growing up. Her mother was very unstable and left the family when she was young. In her subconscious mind, this young woman wanted desperately to have children so that she could indirectly correct or redeem the poor upbringing she had as a child, thereby healing the wounds left by her mother's instability, lack of presence and love. This sort of "mixed" bag of desires became confusing and offsetting for her husband. There was a hidden, subconscious agenda that the woman was bringing to the table of having children, so that it wasn't "their" enterprise together, it was her desires and her agenda that needed to be fulfilled, and so he wasn't really a partner on equal footing in the enterprise of conception, he was just fulfilling a role for her needs. Not every person feels comfortable with that sort of mixed energetic intention, even if the unhealthy desire is not expressed and remains subconscious. It just doesn't feel right and it didn't feel right to him either. It was only when she came to realize the hidden agenda that she had, and began really working on clearing the wounds of her past, that the woman and her husband could have children naturally and in a healthy fashion.

Who knows how these subtle dynamics work? The husband was unsure about having children. That is how it appeared to be at face value to the woman. But when she recognized that her desire was both healthy and natural, as well as unhealthy and coming from a wound, and she worked on that, and let go of that aspect of her need, it became much easier for him to decide. Her anger and frustration toward his indecision reflected the fact that he was frustrating her agenda to redeem herself and her wounded childhood via having children (this is a form of compensation also and is not a healthy dynamic to having children). Was his issue of being a father also a true issue for him to work through? Or did her letting go open up the situation, enabling him to feel more comfortable with having a shared enterprise together? The answer is, it depends, and like the situation, it was likely a mixed bag all happening at the same time.

Chapter 15

Real Situation vs Perceived Situation/Delusion

At times, the difference between a real situation versus a perceived situation may be important to help a patient discern what is really going on. In a real situation, there is a problem that really exists in the world outside the patient's mind and the solution calls for it to be dealt with externally, i.e. in the actual world itself. In a perceived situation, it is more of a personal illusion/delusion that lives inside the person's mind and imagination. This issue calls for an internal adjustment to be made and the outside world should be left alone. Trouble arises when we mistake one for the other.

For example, I had a case of a woman who felt her boss was looking at her like a piece of meat. She felt incredibly uncomfortable around him. Every time she had to go to his office, she felt an extraordinary amount of self-consciousness, like he was undressing her with his eyes. She decided to deal with this for years by believing that the issue was her own problem and it was not really happening. During our appointments, she became aware that she often "takes the blame" on herself, and doesn't trust her own instincts in certain situations. With this awareness, she was able to return to the boss situation, and perceive it for what it was. That he truly was predatory and was undressing her with his eyes. Her feelings had been correct. So it was a real situation that she had mistaken as a perceived situation/delusion.

When a person mistakes a real situation for a perceived situation and blames themselves, they are undermining the very God-given sense of discernment and right and wrong that exists inside of them. This is a big problem also in the New Age world, because everything must be positive and meant to be, and due to the all-pervasiveness of *The Secret* in New Age culture, if there is a problem, the problem must lie inside of me because I am manifesting it. Whereas this is true, sometimes, perhaps often, one needs to discern when it is not, and deal with it accordingly. For this patient, she had to set her boundaries and call him out on his inappropriate behavior.

It does turn out that she also has issues with men, especially aggressive, predatory types. However, first things first. Is her perception of him looking at her like a piece of meat true or just perceived/delusion? It is true. Ok. Then what? Well, then she has to set her boundaries, speak up, deal with it. But she has issues setting her own boundaries with men like that. Aha! Now that is different. One step at a time. First she acknowledged her own feelings were correct. Then, through the Vis Dialogue, I helped her face and deal with her issues surrounding men and setting boundaries, which would start with something like this; *"What makes it difficult for you to set boundaries with men like that?"*

Imagine another situation that is somewhat reversed. A woman has a history of sexual abuse by men. She is highly mistrustful of men. One day, she goes into her boss' office and he comments on how lovely she is looking, in a very benign, complimentary way, but she interprets it as him coming onto her and transgressing her boundaries. She files for sexual harassment. Here, the problem does not live in the world outside, but inside the woman, due to her wound. Yes, the wounding originally did come from the outside, through abuse. But now, the reality of the situation is that she is living in the past and projecting her wound onto other men in her life. This must be dealt with accordingly – i.e., inside of her, and not projected onto them.

Now there is another situation that can occur and it is that, due to a past real situation, for example, sexual abuse, a person adopts a subconscious belief that they are good for nothing else besides being abused, and they can and do continue to attract abusive men into their life, or perhaps be attracted to abusive types. The initial wound was real, but the adopted belief is not, and it is this adopted belief that needs to be addressed and healed so that the repeated unhealthy repetitive patterns can stop.

Chapter 16

The Metaphor of the Mountain Climber

This metaphor combines a situation that involves both a real situation and a perceived situation/delusion during the very same process. For example, a mountain climber is hiking up a mountain with a heavy backpack, laden down with weight. It's a hot day and the sun is baking the mountain climber. All of this is true. It's a real situation and it is a real challenge. The climber will need rest, shade, and good food and water to cover the basics of their body's needs. But, at the same time, the mountain climber starts to think various thoughts that are unnecessary and are all going on inside of their head/imagination that begin to make the already difficult situation worse. "What if I twist my ankle now and fall into the ditch? Who will find me? What if no one finds me?" "What if I run out of water and I die of thirst? Who is going to miss me?" "Why did I come out here all alone? Why don't I have friends or a partner that wants to be here with me? I am so lonely. This isn't fun out here on my own." "What if, what if..."

I have found that the added element of negativity within a situation that has a real challenge is often much worse than the challenge itself. Human beings can accomplish great feats. A mountain climber can do the same. With steady focus, being very present and in the moment and with some toughness and grit, a mountain can be tackled without too much fuss. But when the doubts, fears, self-attack and other issues get inside of the situation, it quickly throws the person out of their center. And it is being outside one's center that makes them susceptible to injury and disease.

For example, I have some cases of people who have very difficult lives. They are working two, sometimes three or more jobs to make ends meet for their family, all the while being single parents. In time, with some good healing of negative mindsets and expectations of suffering and of life being hard, along with good strategies and planning, this real and tough situation can change. But in the meantime, there is no way out. This is it. A really tough and really real situation. It has its challenge in and of itself. And it is causing suffering and disease. So how do you help such a patient? The only way you can help them, is to find what perceived/delusions or inner doubts, fears, and other internal beliefs are piggy-backing inside of this already difficult situation. Sometimes, that is enough to help change the situation. At the very least, like the challenge of the mountain climber, they will be able to handle the tough times if they are centered, present, and living in their heart. If they doubt, oppose, or question themselves, it makes it much, much worse, even to the point of it being intolerable. In my cases of patients who have carried tremendous loads on their backs, I have helped them in the only way I can – by helping them recognize what is unnecessary that is going on inside of the real situation. It is often fear, and self-doubt. "Can I handle this on my own?" "What if I can't continue to do this? What will happen to my family?" The power of fear and doubt are debilitating enough to make any do-able challenge almost impossible. If the mountain climber's backpack weighs 40 pounds, with the doubt and fear, it becomes as if it were 200 pounds. In such cases, I would ask questions to investigate what is being carried that is unnecessary.

Chapter 17

Things Seeming to Get Worse When They are Really Getting Better

I have observed in my practice an odd phenomenon where patients complain of feeling as if they were getting worse when they are clearly getting better. The client's Shen ("light in the eyes" energy) is stronger. Their pulse is better. They are digesting and eliminating their food better. Their overall countenance is better, yet from their perspective, they perceive themselves as getting worse. The simplest way to explain this is, "Ignorance is bliss." Before they begin healing, or before any sort of self-awareness, people are shut-down and completely out of touch with themselves, so the amount of pain they experience is next to nothing. It's like they are frozen and unaware of their pain and the dysfunction of their subconscious self. As they begin their healing process, they begin to open up areas inside of themselves that are quite painful. As this continues, the healed self becomes ever more conscious of that which is still out of balance or wounded, and so the relative awareness of the suffering increases, all the while that the healing is bringing about an improvement in health and a decrease of the amount of blocked and unhealthy energy in their system. I have heard a few patients tell me, somewhat seriously, so I had to refrain from laughing at how comical it sounded, "Doctor, I used to feel happy before I came to see you." These patients had begun dealing with some very unhappy situations and unhealthy aspects of themselves that they were blissfully ignorant of before we began working together. And that is the way in which some patients express their gratitude at how much you're helping them face the light. "You made me miserable, doctor!"

As we discussed layers of consciousness, the older the layer, the more deeply buried and the more potent the issues are buried. So, the beginning of one's healing journey may be the easiest. Beliefs that no longer serve are peeled away with ease, and the person walks down the sidewalk jumping and clinking their heels together. But as long as they are willing to progress down through the depths of their psyche, the challenges do get more difficult and intense. Each subsequent "victory" in healing and progress is also that much more liberating and cause for celebration. It also prepares one for the deeper and more difficult challenges that lie ahead. In this way, also, a person can have the impression that things are getting worse, when they are really getting better, especially when they are in the thick of things on a deeper level. This may need to be explained to some people, especially if they are resenting you for "ruining their life." And the healing itself can be quite up and down, as one gets extremely challenged during the healing only to feel tremendous release, relief, and joy at breaking through a given layer.

Another phenomenon which closely resembles this topic is the idea that there needs to be a brief loss of control over that which the patient has controlled or over that which has controlled them, before there is a major improvement. So if a patient has been controlling and burying their anger, some loss of control over their anger is necessary to bring about a healing. If a patient has been "locking themselves down" so they never lose control in public in order to not embarrass themselves, there needs to be some form of loss of this control as well in order to progress on their healing. This loss of control is experienced by the patient as a worsening of their state, since they have mandated themselves to not lose control. Yet this worsening of the situation is only an *apparent* worsening. Things are actually moving in the right direction. This is akin to the homeopathic aggravation, where things can seem to be getting worse before they improve. And here, too, the term aggravation in homeopathy is at times a misnomer, because it is only the unhealthy elements that are being released. However, they can bring about a sense of worsening of the situation for the patient before the feeling of catharsis. This is in total contrast when comparing to how symptoms are immediately suppressed and falsely "improved" in allopathic treatment. Patients need to be brought to an understanding of this topic so that they can appreciate the phenomena they are experiencing as positive and encouraging, rather than dissuasive and as a reason to run back to the quick fix of allopathy.

There is another situation where a person must let go of control before healing can occur and that is during possessions by unwanted entities. When a person's body, mind, or emotions have been taken over in any way, at the time the entity is "cast out," there is a momentary loss of control where the entity will seem to take over completely and the person experiences a total loss of control. It must first rise up so that it can go out. Imagine a creature lurking at the bottom of a lake. This is the lake of the subconscious. If we want it out of our subconscious, it must first surface. As it surfaces, it conveys an impression that it is taking over, but it is not. It is really only this phenomenon that I am discussing now that is occurring – that which has controlled is being released. It brings with it the sense of loss of control. This must occur for healing to happen.

Chapter 18

The Intolerance of Time and Repetition

Earlier in the chapter on *Errors in Innocence*, I explained how the consequences of making a mistake becomes more and more dire with each subsequent "slip" back into the addictive behavior, compensation or substance. This happens more once there is awareness surrounding the mistake, and even if there is not awareness. *The Intolerance of Time and Repetition* is this very same phenomenon. If a patient asks, "Why is it that every time I go against what is good for me, the consequences become worse?" You can, as a practitioner, ask a question, "*What do you think the answer is?*" I like to do that and then confirm with the patient if their understanding is accurate. Or, if they need a little help, to assist them in coming to the understanding they feel most in alignment with. Sometimes, even if I wanted to, I don't have an answer for them. So I ask them the question, hoping they'll come up with something wise and resolve their own question.

Like an addict who decides to have a fix after being clean for a while, the consequences become more and more dire with each subsequent "slip" back into their addictive substance. The same is true for belief systems and compensation patterns. For example, a woman tends to be attracted to older men that don't treat her well and that serves both having someone to look up to because she doesn't have much self-esteem and also fits because she is also punishing herself, because she doesn't feel good about herself. When she recognizes what is underlying this pattern for her and yet she chooses to be with another man who fits the same pattern, it will have the worst consequences she has ever seen. The reason for this is a bit of a mystery but it is nevertheless true. I can surmise that it is because the Universe actually does want the best for us, and when we follow a way of compensation and fear, it gets tougher on us, in order to push us in the right direction. Our own consciousness, as being connected through the soul to the Creator, must also be involved in this principle.

This phenomenon does not only coincide with slips in addictive substances or relationships, i.e. it is not always related to something external. It can really be a slip back into a belief system. If a person has been free of a belief for a while, and has "seen through it" only to fall into it again, giving it the credence as if it is true and real, the consequences will become worse each time. It's like our being has less tolerance for the false belief as we continue to let it go and then re-choose it again, like we are getting impatient with ourselves and the pressure is being upped.

This can resemble how in truly embedded beliefs, each subsequent time we encounter that belief in ourselves also represents our facing a deeper degree of the belief. Earlier encounters of the belief were easier to chip away, but as the belief is encountered at its deeper level, it represents a more difficult challenge to liberate. This coincides with the phenomenon of *things seeming to be getting worse when they are really getting better*, because a person is actually in a healthier state following becoming more aware of themselves. Things are better, yet with a slip that comes further on during the process of healing, it will bring with it a stronger challenge to the patient. However, it is different if the belief or the unhealthy pattern is truly gone and then it is "re-chosen," there is less tolerance for it with each subsequent embrace and the patient will have a much more difficult time liberating themselves each time it is "re-chosen." In this way, time is intolerant of repetition in healing.

Chapter 19

No Room for Any More – Sympathetic Resonance

There is a celestial mind-force, a great sympathetic force which is life itself, of which everything is composed. John Keely

In this Universe, similar frequencies resonate with each other. A tuning fork of the same note, when tapped, will cause another tuning fork of the same note/frequency, to resonate, even though the two are separated by some distance. This is a law called *The Law of Sympathetic Vibration*.[13] The same is true for emotion. Sadness resonates with sadness. Jealousy with jealousy. Joy with joy. Sexual energy with sexual energy. The more similar the emotion, the more it will trigger or, cause to resonate, the other similar emotion. For instance, sadness over the loss of a child that is carried by the parents who feel guilty and as if they should have done more to save their child, will resonate very strongly with the same in others, and not quite as much with someone who lost a child but knew there was nothing they could do. The sadness will resonate with the sadness. The sadness about the loss of the child will resonate even more strongly with the sadness about the loss of the child, and then the guilt therein, will add even more resonance.

When we work with patients, their stuck and wounded emotions will cause our own stuck and wounded emotions to resonate. This is another reason that "Physician, Heal Thyself!" is so vital. The idea of something causing something else to resonate is the same as saying that something "triggers" something else. And now we can explain better as to why that is. This is a fascinating topic and one that could be expanded upon quite a lot. One can also read *John Keely's Law of Sympathetic*

128

Vibration by Dale Pond to learn more about the science surrounding this phenomenon.

What else does this have to do with practice? I have noticed a person that has an unhealthy issue with a certain type of energy, will have no more room to be around or to face a similar issue in the world until they become aware and heal themselves. For example, I have seen many cases where people would like to avoid responsibility in their lives. Anything that brings more responsibility is avoided. At first glance, the person may simply seem to have an issue with responsibility. But why? The answer often lies in the fact that they are already carrying a heavy and unhealthy responsibility, so, by the "law of sympathetic vibration" they simply have no more room for any more responsibility. It is also that any other responsibility resonates with their own unhappy, unhealthy responsibility and makes them uncomfortable, thus, they wish to avoid the situation or endeavor that triggers the inner issue. For example, one man that I was working with in his late twenties had a lot of issues with having a job, and getting married. Upon investigation, the issues he was having with both were the same – it was about the responsibility. He wanted to avoid it. Upon further investigation, it became clear that as a young child, he began to feel responsible for the well-being of his parents. This is not uncommon for many young adults to carry around a feeling of responsibility for the well-being of their parents. Some of these young adults will have little room for more responsibility, because more responsibility stacks up on the back of the other unhealthy responsibility. The thought that a child is responsible for the well-being of their parents is unhealthy and, I may add, untrue. Each person is responsible for their own well-being, except for children who have to be taken care of until a certain age. A person can have many healthy responsibilities and feel fine, but when one carries an unhealthy responsibility, there is no room for more, even healthy, responsibilities, because responsibility resonates with/triggers responsibility. Whoa, that was a lot of the word responsibility in one sentence.

As another example:

In one case, where I got down to the bottom line with a person and asked, *"Do you want to continue living this way?"* They wanted to say no and to change, but they had a major blockage and were really resisting making that change. With some investigation, we discovered that, as a child, she had often had to move from town to town, state to state. Every year, my patient had to change schools, cities, and friends. This was extremely hard on her. But because she had grown up feeling responsible for her parents' well-being, she did not voice any of those difficult feelings she had surrounding change. So, she felt change meant feeling bad but not being able to voice it because she felt responsible to protect her parents from feeling anything negative coming from her. So for her, even in something seemingly completely unrelated, when I asked her if she wanted to continue living this way, she didn't want to say yes, because change represented an unhappy place of unexpressed feelings and more unhappy, unhealthy responsibility. Getting to the bottom of this did actually help her recognize what was making her resist the change, and so she was then able to say, "No. I do not want to live this way any longer," and she moved on with her life to begin to really improve beyond that particular belief that was inhibiting her.

In this case, change (good, positive) resonated with the change in her which had been unhappy and unhealthy. So, even something good and healthy can trigger/resonate with something of the like nature that has a wounded negative connotation surrounding it. Male energy resonates with male energy. People, often women, who have had bad experiences with the male energy in men, be it physical, sexual, or verbal abuse, will have a hard time being around even healthy male energy in others because it resonates with the troubling male energy that wounded them. Naturally, a strong, abusive man will resonate more with the source of the wounds of their own abuse than a healthy, strong man, but most who have been wounded by an aggressive, strong male energy will have a strong reaction and either react and push away (energetically or literally), try to suppress in turn, or try to avoid the healthy, strong male energy and not be able to be around it. There is no room for any of it. A person wounded by the unhealthy male energy in others will likely divorce themselves from their own male energy. One of the positive and healthy aspects in the male energy is discernment, so a person who is wounded by unhealthy male energy will divorce themselves from discernment, the one energy they need to discern the difference between the healthy male and the unhealthy male energy. Ironic, isn't it?

Boundaries sympathetically resonate with boundaries. A person who has unhealthy boundaries and who is accustomed to not honoring their own boundaries will have no room for a connection with healthy boundaries with someone else. They will often not want to have any more relationships other than the ones they have already established with the unhealthy boundaries, because unhealthy boundaries leave no room for any form of relationships requiring boundaries of any sort (healthy or unhealthy). Hence the "no room for any more." This can be helpful to keep in mind during practice.

Chapter 20

What is the Difference between an Exciting Cause and The Root Cause?

An exciting cause is a trigger that brings on the symptoms or brings forward a flare-up or manifestation of a disease, but is not the underlying or root cause of the disease. For example, eating wheat can cause a flare-up of the symptoms of many conditions, like eczema, Celiac disease, IBS, even anxiety. Some would say, "wheat causes my disease" instead of saying, wheat is an exciting cause of the disease. In Celiac, even if it is a genetically inherited condition, something else has led to the disposition of the disease in the first place, which is its true and underlying, root cause. As another example, a boy's epileptic seizures are triggered around high tension wires. Some would say, the EMFs (electromagnetic fields) are causing his seizures, and it wouldn't be entirely incorrect, only that the EMFs are an exciting cause, and not the root cause, which could be any number of things. Sugar can be an exciting cause of migraines, but it is not the root cause, which could be any number of mental-emotional issues.

By eliminating the exciting cause, the disease is not cured, but rather, controlled. If that exciting cause is reintroduced, then the patient will have a return of their symptoms. But when a root cause is removed, the disease is cured and will not come back even if the person is exposed to an exciting cause.

If a condition is truly caused by an environmental factor, such as a low form of illness caused by living in a swamp, or regularly drinking water with a high level of toxicity, or living next to an electrical power plant, or working at a terrible job, the cause of the illness is limited to the exposure of the exciting cause. Removing the exciting cause removes all traces of the condition which means that the condition has no root cause, but is only brought on by the conditional exposure to an unhealthy environment. Change the environment and the person improves. This shows that it is not a chronic condition, but more of an acute condition, or an indisposition which will be ameliorated by removal from the disturbing environmental factor. One can gain some insight into the picture of the "whole person," however, by observing which areas of the body are first and most affected. In a swamp, does a person begin getting low back pain or do their knees begin to ache and swell? When someone is in a difficult, stressful, unhealthy job, which organ systems or body parts are first and most affected? This sort of susceptibility, which gives a place for unhealthy environmental factors to take effect and cause problems, points more to the root cause in the individual or at least to the source of the susceptibility inside the person. The weakness in the given system or body part, when explored, would give rise to a feeling, sensation, or picture that would point toward the underlying belief system that is out of harmony that has thrown the emotional field and the body out of balance, leaving it susceptible to injury and influence by environmental factors. When young children fall down steep hills, they often fall down floppily and rise at the bottom unscathed. When adults fall down the same sort of hill, however, they will sustain injury. Where they are injured is often an indication of where they have a lot of tension and rigidity in their body. The tension and rigidity in the body points to a place in the mental-emotional realms that is also rigid and tense. Any injury that the adult sustains in such a fall that becomes chronic will also need to be addressed at the root cause of the injury – namely, in the mental beliefs that resonate with and have led that body part to reflect its rigid and tense belief. There are more factors in chronic injury which we will take a look at in Chapter 30 of this book.

Chapter 21

Addressing Obstacles to Cure in Practice

Even though we understand that there is a root cause in the mind, which then translates into the emotional field and becomes manifest in the body, there are times when a case of chronic illness cannot be cured because there are obstacles standing in the way. When a practitioner addresses the root cause of a chronic illness and the patient is not recovering, something may be blocking the Vital Force. A thorough investigation needs to be conducted to try to determine what the obstacle to cure may be. It may be a strongly negative environmental factor, as we just mentioned. For example, a person has migraines, and upon diving deeply through the Vis Dialogue, it becomes clear that the person is always worrying because they feel if they don't worry, bad things are going to happen. So the belief is the root cause, and it is addressed, but the headaches are not quite going away. Something else is being repeatedly introduced into the patient's system that is not allowing the Vital Force to recover and restore the system to balance and harmony. Upon investigation, you discover that the patient is eating 10 boxes of Kraft Dinner per week and they are sensitive to the artificial flavours in the product. Removing this obstacle can allow the body to recover and remove the migraines from their system. The Kraft dinner could have also been an exciting cause in the case and it could have been bringing on the migraines at times. But since the patient had begun getting migraines even before they had ever first eaten Kraft Dinner, or anything of the like, we know the root cause to be in the negative beliefs they have and the obstacle to cure to be inside of the Kraft Dinner. We can also say that a body may not be healed of its root cause when the exciting cause is continuously introduced.

I had a case of myasthenia gravis where the patient, following our first appointment, was making a lot of changes in her life and had begun to improve a lot on her outlook and her overall mental-emotional disposition. Yet the severe ptosis in her right eye had not improved at all. During our first follow-up, upon investigation of her symptoms, she described them as being "draining and frustrating" and they made her feel very negative. I asked if there was anywhere else in her life that made her feel this way. This is a Holistic Counseling technique designed to bridge between a patient's symptoms and their life, which I share in more detail later. She replied that yes, she had a few friends that made her feel that way. Her story was that she had two friends in particular that would call her and complain for hours on end. When I asked for clarification, she said that yes, she meant it literally. She would spend between 3-6 hours *per day* listening to them complain and go on and on about very negative details regarding their lives. Day after day this was going on and she said it felt draining to her and she was very frustrated about it. And there is a reflection in the present manifestation of her symptoms. She used the same three words to describe both the situation with her friends and her symptoms, which is a clear indication that they are related. I asked her which ear she held the phone to and she said her right ear – right adjacent to her right eye. And she was using an iPhone 4. IPhones are known to have very high levels of radiation. So not only was she exposing herself to very high levels of damaging radiation from her cell phone, she was also forcing herself to sit there and be drained and annoyed by very negative complaints of her friends. It was like making a negative mixture of two very unhealthy energies. We explored this and she was ready to make a change both in her friend situation and in how long she was going to use her cell phone each day. I know this was not the root cause of her illness, because her symptoms clearly began surrounding an issue she had with an ex-boyfriend. Following our initial consultation, she had improved her outlook toward him (an ex-boyfriend who was recently deceased) and had already begun to feel better about it… but without any changes in her ocular symptoms, something was blocking her! And it was the cell phone use as well as the nature of the conversations she was subjecting herself to.

Other obstacles to cure can be cigarette smoke, recreational drug use, pharmaceutical drugs, exposure to toxic environmental factors, sick houses, GMO foods, history of vaccinations, and many other possibilities. There may also be more than one obstacle to cure in a given case. When a case should be improving but is not, we need to investigate, explore, discover, and address.

Chapter 22

Rightful Action for Correction

First, it is important to share that healing occurs on many levels. Just as an old proverb of unknown origin states – The Thought becomes the Word becomes the Deed becomes the Habit becomes the Character – so too does the healing begin with the change in thought, which is then expressed through the word, which is then brought into action. Eventually, this becomes habit and then is so integrated into one's character, that it is a no-brainer, part of the self, no need for thinking, or choosing. It's a done deal. The healing takes full effect, however, becomes truly set into motion not with the thought or with the word, but once the person has taken the *rightful action* that is a reflection of their healed state. It's a most excellent start for me to recognize that I don't need to be the best to be ok with myself. It's then great for me to share this through my word with myself and my friends and loved ones. "You know, I don't need to be the best anymore. I am fine with the way I am." But if, at the first opportunity when someone comes along that I feel threatened by and that I feel I need to be better than, I forget my thought and my word and fall back into normal needing to be the best behavior, then the healing has not taken place. It could look like me staying up at night worrying about them being better than me. It could also look like me trying to beat them in everything they do, or prove I am better by walking better, talking better, dressing better, getting better grades if I am in school, or making better sales if that is my job. The thought and word have begun a change, but the real healing is not complete until the action is corrected. It is when I truly stop the behavior associated with the unhealthy state and change my action in the world that my healing takes place. So that would look like me not even worrying about it.

Doing my own thing. Accepting them for their greatness and not applying any action to try to be the best in relation to them or anyone else. Then, through the action, the most healing energies flow and restore the person back to their optimal health.

Having established that, we can explore this idea from another perspective. In some cases, a change in the outside world will bring about healing. However, sometimes it does not. Somewhat like the earlier chapter on *Real or Perceived* problems, it all depends on what the action of change is accomplishing. Let's explore the difference.

In one case, a woman is in an unhealthy marriage. She is sick with rheumatoid arthritis (RA). She does not leave because she feels that she is not worthy of living a happy life. Then finally, she gains the courage and leaves the relationship. And then her RA improves and completely resolves. Her leaving is a healthy action for her. It represents her loving herself more and not settling for the idea and action that she is not worthy of living a happy life.

In another case, another woman with rheumatoid arthritis is in an unhappy marriage. She is constantly irritated by her husband and decides to leave him. But it does not improve her RA. Why is that? Because in this second case example, upon further exploration, it becomes clear that this woman believes that people should do everything according to her wishes, and when her husband was not complying, she became extremely irritated with him. But then she chose not express her anger and irritation because she believed that her anger made her less than perfect. So her healing would involve her changing her belief systems – both that the expression of anger means one is not perfect, but even more importantly for her, to let go of the thought that people should do everything in the way she wishes. Then she can speak to her husband when he does something that is not according to her wishes by saying, "That's ok. You don't have to do it exactly the way I say." And finally, the rightful action is not getting mad and loving her husband regardless of how he is being and what she wants. Eventually, with enough healed thoughts, words, and actions, it won't even cross her mind that he has done something to annoy her because it wasn't what she had wanted. It won't elicit anger, and so there won't even be any anger to suppress. Eventually, she may be able to get mad at him legitimately when he does something that is truly boundary crossing or upsetting to her, and that will be a healthy form of expression for her.

For one person, leaving an unhealthy job brings about a complete recovery, whereas, for a different person, leaving their job does nothing to improve their condition. In the first case, the person's true nature is being restricted and it is simply a hostile environment where the unhealthy factors exist outside themselves. So a change in the environment represents a good action. In the second example, the problem lives inside of the person. They never speak up or stick up for themselves and they go from one job to the next where they are continuously dominated and taken advantage of because they don't speak up or stand up for themselves. Their rightful action must come from within them and their environment does not have to change to do so. In fact, when they change their inner environment and begin taking rightful action by speaking up and standing up for themselves, they will find that their outer environment changes to reflect their own inside. This will often happen and as a result, health and happiness follow. Now, it can also occur that they do change their inner environment but people continue to treat them in a fashion that is not conducive to how they are truly and newly feeling about themselves. Their outer environment is unable to meet their own changed inner environment, despite their own healthy and rightful action. This would then become as in the first case example where a person leaves their unhealthy environment and that is their rightful action.

In short, when there is no issue within, changing an unhealthy environment will bring about positive effects on one's health and well-being. If the change needs to take place from within, changing one's external environment to "get away" from it, will not bring about any positive change. There are some New Age teachings, like *The Secret*, that make it seem as if everything that happens in a person's environment is a reflection of them. I have found that this is simply not always the case. It can confuse a person to stay in an unhealthy environment when it is not a reflection of them but simply of the environment or the people in the environment and so the distinction is important to find a balance.

Part III

The Vis Dialogue of Holistic Counseling

The Dialogue of Holistic Counseling can be simply called the Vis Dialogue. The word Vis comes from the Latin phrase *Vis Medicatrix Naturae*, meaning The Healing Power of Nature. Naturopaths often simply use the word The Vis to abridge this principle of Naturopathic medicine.

The purpose of the Vis Dialogue is to reveal the underlying cause of a person's illness/problem and to then help them unchoose it and release it. In other words, it's to help a person see (*doctor as teacher*) what their problem is and to help them see how to change it. Another way to look at the purpose of the Vis Dialogue is to challenge what a patient believes. It is to get them to consider that some of the choices they're making may not be in their best interest. However, the practitioner is not in a mindset to be pushing aggressively to get a patient's defenses up, but rather, to be asking questions that serve to challenge the validity (as measured up to the Universal Truth and a person's I AM) of the patient's beliefs.

It is a most simple method. This does not mean it is easy. However, by simply applying a few principles in practice, much progress can be done with a case to help people profoundly.

The simple elements of the method of Holistic Counseling are as follows:

Ask non-directive questions.

Follow the stream – ask the next question based on the last thing a person said.

Keep going deeper into the rabbit hole until the root cause is discovered.

Then help the patient reflect where this root cause came from and,

Recognize that it is not something that is serving them.

Then help the patient recognize the choice they have to make and ask them if they wish to continue living that way.

Then celebrate with them when they are ready to change.

That's it. The rest is commentary and how to deal with difficult and exceptional situations.

Chapter 23

Attitude of the Practitioner

I have found the attitude of the practitioner to best serve the practice when the practitioner is calm, friendly, easy-going, and lighthearted. It may be a good way to remind the patient that despite the intensity of their own experience, everything is ultimately alright. This is just an attitude and it is not something that one is trying to "teach" the patient. In other words, by being easy-going, we are not trying to say "lighten up!" Avoiding being too serious is a good idea, unless matching the state of the patient. If a patient is struck with deep grief, matching the energy of that sort of mood is important.

One important attitude to also completely stay clear from is a "know-it-all" sort of attitude. This creates a dynamic that is counter-intuitive for the idea the practitioner is endeavoring to impart to the patient – that the answers for their own questions already live inside of them as they emanate from the Vis. In one seminar that I took with Rajans Sankaran, the India homeopath and author, he told us he likes to appear "stupid and lazy" in practice. The idea is that when his patients perceive him being so, they work harder to tell him what he needs to know, rather than when he appeared to be very intelligent and all-knowing, they didn't tell him much at all, believing, rather, that he possessed all the answers himself and needed nothing from them. I am not suggesting to make oneself appear stupid and lazy. Just don't appear to know it all.

I like to prepare before every dialogue/consultation by opening my heart and remembering to be tuned in to the person's highest good. Setting this intention can only take a brief moment or longer if desired. I tap in to remind myself of what I am doing, and what I am there for. I commit to being present, even when I am not feeling very good. This helps me get into the moment and get absorbed into the dialogue. It usually never fails that within a short amount of time, my own troubles or discomfort in myself are alleviated and I am totally immersed in the good feelings that come from being totally present for someone else's well-being. It is especially important for me to prepare these intentions before appointments with patients that are challenging and difficult and that put my compassion to the test. If I do not prepare my intention, it is easier for me to get frustrated with how challenging they can be, rather than being filled with a feeling of compassion, which is a good lubricant that helps to oil even the most troubling and obstinate engines.

I have found being open in mind, emotion, and heart to be one of the most important ways of practicing Holistic Counseling. Being open is a natural consequence of being healed and feeling ok with oneself. Being healed is not an absolute state of being, but rather a continuum toward an ever-evolving state of well-being. Openness in the practitioner encourages openness in the patient. Being shut down emotionally may be the very least productive state for practicing Holism, as the patient will undoubtedly sense a shut-down state in the practitioner and will not feel comfortable being exposed and vulnerable. It is somewhat akin to having to take off your clothes in front of people who are all dressed. One feels put on the spot and judged.

Another important aspect of the attitude of the practitioner involves being non-judgmental. This, like being open, is not so much an act of effort, as it is a result of going through one's own healing process. When we go through our own wounds and get to encounter the resultant ego that is built up to remain in control over the wound, we realize how very difficult and trying an endeavor it really is. This helps to crystallize in our mind how each of us has our dark side, our wound that at times is beyond our control, and how easy it is to "fall" in this life. This garners humility in a practitioner which is an important companion to non-judgmentalness. There are people who go through life thinking there is nothing wrong with them and that everyone should just "get over" their problems and move on. They do not realize that they are operating from within their ego and their attitude is not emerging from a true place but rather from an illusory place where they feel they need to be invulnerable, likely as a compensatory mechanism for how vulnerable and small they really feel. There is an Israeli expression that says (transliterated) "Rofeh tov holech le gehenom," which translates as "A good doctor goes through hell." And it is true that a doctor that has gone through their own "dark side," their own hell, is prepared for helping others through their suffering.

Being totally present and being a good listener is also of great importance. The ability to "set aside" oneself is key to a successful practice. We all get into difficult times. Sometimes those stresses and worries are easy to take home and to carry around with us. It is important to be able to step out of ourselves to focus on the words, thoughts, and feelings of another. This is another way that practicing holistically is very healing, because it demonstrates the fact that those issues we were dwelling on, that seemed so pervasive and real, couldn't have been all that vital since we just spent one hour completely forgetting all about them. It reaffirms the smallness of the issues while helping to remind ourselves that we are ultimately ok, no matter what has been troubling us. The candle staring meditation that I share in class is an excellent exercise to train the mind to be focused on one point and to be able to tune into something else besides one's own present needs.

It is greatly important to be patient in practice. Don't rush it. Don't force people to get to it already. Give people the time they need to express themselves. Stay with a person and know that they will slowly open up even if they didn't at first. I once had a case that I felt was going around and around in circles for close to one hour. I felt I wasn't getting anywhere. The patient was answering with only the very minor and superficial reflection into themselves. Their mind was strongly built up in defense to not see the inner wound beyond the story they had told themselves of being totally fine, having it all figured out, not needing anyone's help. If I had been a beginner during this case, I would have likely given up, but I had seen other cases like this that didn't seem to be getting anywhere suddenly turn around with a new and different angle or question, or sometimes, just the same question repeated following a series of other questions. It's like loosening a knot. Sometimes we have to tug at a few different points of the rope surrounding the knot until it loosens. This particular patient had built up so much resistance to being in touch with themselves, that it took literally close to one hour of questions, until their knot loosened and they began to rapidly and deeply cycle through the questions, moving quickly toward the root of their problem as it lay in their subconscious.

Lacking patience often lies as a problem for many beginner practitioners. They think to themselves, "I've got to get them deeper. I've got to get to the core." For whatever reason, some lack of confidence in themselves, some struggle with being too in control and needing to make it happen for the patient. Beginners haven't had the necessary experience to see, time and time again, how the patient will get there given enough time. Some patients, perhaps the more self-aware ones, get there sooner, whereas others can take up to between one half hour and one hour to even begin the process of answering questions in a deeper and deeper fashion toward uncovering their underlying core-limiting and dis-ease creating belief. So, for now, take my word for it. It's going to happen. Take your time. Give it time and give them time. They will get to it, even if it is not during one session, but at the next one. There are exercises and homework you can give to facilitate a breakthrough, which I will discuss later. In time, as you see the bud of a person's mind open during a Vis Dialogue, you will gain experience that turns into trusting the process over time and much experience. Eventually, that trust and confidence will build on itself, and is an attractive balm to the sick and the suffering.

A trust is formed toward the practitioner when the practitioner is a good listener and asks good questions. People often have never spoken to anyone about the issues they are sharing with the practitioner and many have never even thought of reflecting on the questions you ask them in the Vis Dialogue. When you get a person to say, "Good question!" you know you have engaged them. It is a sign you can relax (if you haven't already) and you can trust that they are now "all ears" so to speak. When a person says, "Good question!" in that reverent sort of way, they are also saying, "Wow, I have never thought of that before. That is a very valuable question that is getting me to reflect on some very important things in my life." And they are right! The value of the right question is beyond measure.

In terms of practice management, patients that have those aha moments and "Good question!" proclamations are most likely to return to your practice. Earlier in my practice, there were periods of time where I relied strictly on my skill as a homeopath. As is natural with beginner homeopaths and even for some seasoned homeopaths during difficult cases, the remedies would not act for the first, second, and even sometimes up to third or fourth remedy selection. It was then that the patients were not coming back to the greatest degree. But now that I use Holistic Counseling in all of my cases, those patients who have had aha and "Good question!" moments, almost always come back, and when they don't, it's usually because they are doing very well and I have become obsolete in their life. So in those cases that I haven't quite fully perceived the homeopathic remedy they need, they have gotten some greatly relevant healing from the Holistic Counseling that makes them feel they are getting a lot out of our interactions. This brings them back and it also takes pressure off the practitioner to "find the right remedy," an element of practice that can be challenging for many homeopaths and Naturopathic doctors.

Being patient and allowing the case to unravel is a fundamentally important attitude of the practitioner, and it must be balanced with the knowing that the practitioner is in charge. People can go on and on by telling a story that doesn't go any deeper than the surface of the story with all its details. As a practitioner, don't allow them to go around and around, or on and on. Some people will do this if given the space. So, have a guidance in your mind, an intention, to get to the cause. People love to be listened to. It can be therapeutic for them just to be listened to, but it is not purposeful to just sit and be the listener, if that is the only thing that is happening and no progress of understanding is occurring. It is important to recognize that people can talk without revealing anything of the inner workings of their mental and emotional worlds. It is important to steer people in the right direction, and to bring up the stuff that makes up their problem. It is important for the practitioner to be clear on this, for this particular situation, where a patient is just talking and not revealing anything. It is there that the practitioner needs to be in charge of the direction of the dialogue – not the patient. If you notice that the patient is not going anywhere, they are just avoiding by telling stories, avoiding the issues at hand – then it is important to gently interrupt and bring the focus back toward going deeper and to getting to the cause of illness. When I see this happening, I will say something along the lines of, *"Ok. I can see you feel you have a lot to tell about this story. I can understand that. But in order for me to help you, it's important to get deeper and beyond just the story so that you can answer questions about how the story is actually affecting you."* There is that firmness/male quality that is important during times like this. It is important to get a general idea of the story of a person's life to have a context for the discussion and for going deeper. But when the person keeps going back to telling the story and is not answering from a deeper place, they are avoiding going deeper.

Stopping them and pointing out that it is important to reflect deeper is helpful to progress the case. It is important to note that people often revert to telling the story at the very point in the dialogue where they are about to uncover something painful and core inside of them. This is all the more reason to bring them back to the dialogue, rather than allowing them to evade by jumping back into the story.

Another reason they just tell the story is because they have a strong feeling of not being heard and of needing to be listened to as a result. So, the telling of the story and you listening to it is a means of them fulfilling their need to be listened to. This is not the point of Holistic Counseling, just as the practitioner should never enable the need that emerges from a patient's false reality and wound. So if a person has the feeling they are disrespected, our role is not to make them feel respected by giving them respect, but rather by helping them get to and then release the false ideas surrounding them feeling disrespected. We are not to provide company for the patient that feels lonely and lost in the world, but to help them recreate a healthier reality where that happens spontaneously and equally, where it becomes a non-issue for them. Telling a patient that feels ugly and useless that they are beautiful and very, very needed in the world is allopathic counseling. As a practitioner, giving someone respect or company that feels disrespected or lonely is like providing yourself as the "feel good" drug of the allopathic method. It is ultimately not healthy for patient or practitioner. The same applies for listening to patients that don't feel heard. Get comfortable with the male energy stepping in gently, as balanced with the female, to get them from the surface story to the depths.

Venting for a patient is also therapeutic but only temporarily. You can help your patients feel better, temporarily, by allowing them to vent, but if they return the next time, and they need to vent about the same issue that keeps occurring, how much have you really helped them? So you have to decide if you want to be a shoulder to cry on, or a healer.

Be seamless. Have a seamless dialogue. Be as conversational as possible. Don't make the questioning process obvious, robotic, or "clinical" sounding. Having a smooth flow takes the patient's mind off the obviousness of the setting (exploring healing with questions), and helps to gather momentum for the opening of their subconscious. It is also ok to have some long pauses where a patient reflects, contacts some feelings, cries, gets clear on their issue, and breathes. Holistic Counseling is like playing live Jazz music. As we adlib through the phrasing of the questions and bring up each subsequent question based on the previous answer the patient expressed, there is a rhythm and a constancy to the music. However, in music, there is something called "dynamics," where the song is not always played out at the very same rhythm and intensity. To bring in some quiet spots, "bring it down," rests, pauses, adds a lot of dynamic to the music and helps it from becoming monotonous at always the same rhythm. Often this just happens naturally and doesn't need to be something to which too much attention is given. It's just a beautiful thing to see how a pause, or a rest, can bring about renewed musical energy to the seamless rhythm of the dialogue.

Chapter 24

Be a "Detective" of Nature, Not a Projector!

Our goal is to uncover the cause of illness as it lives within a patient, not to project what we believe is the underlying cause of their illness. Even if you are gifted psychically and you can see what you think is the cause, the good nature doctor helps the patient see it for themselves, as much as possible. This is difficult for a gifted psychic as they may be able to perceive the person's problems. However, after I have practiced Holistic Counseling enough, I can even see the limitation in relation to the amount of healing that can occur that is inherent in telling someone what their problem is through an intuitive/psychic process. It simply does not have enough of the patient's own self-awareness to have a deeply and lastingly transformative effect. And, unfortunately, there are many psychics that, put plainly, are not very accurate. They are not well-trained, do not possess a pure gift, or are just plainly delusional. And how is the patient to really know the difference if the psychic/medium just comes out and tells them what they see, or think they see, is their problem? I have had several cases where a patient conveys to me what a psychic told them about their problem or the cause of their disease. I say, *"Ok, that may be the case, but wouldn't you like to find out for yourself?"* And then, upon some natural, organic, following-the-stream open-ended, non-directional questions, the patient has a complete revelation of what their problem is and can actually see the connection between their illness, their suffering and what they have chosen to believe in their mind. They see it. Often, thinking back to what the psychic said, there is no rapport. They simply were not accurate. I have also seen some psychics and mediums to be quite accurate, impressively so, but another problem emerges and that is "So, now what?" Basically, if a person is told what their problem is but has no connection with the information, so now what? What do they do with it? Holistic Counseling helps a person see the relevance in making the connection between mind and body, between the suffering story and the unhealthy and untrue choices. It goes through all the layers of the house of cards. It helps to unravel a thread from the beginning to the end, so that when it is arrived at (where it starts), the patient has also unravelled it through all the levels and implications that it holds for them. The difference between seeing it themselves and just being told is immeasurable.

I am not attempting to cast an entirely negative shadow over psychics, or medical intuitives because there are times when it can be very useful, and I've sought out their help myself on many occasions. But I do feel in chronic disease, it is best to help a patient see for themselves.

As I will share later in Chapter 27 on the different types of feedback, there are ways of giving feedback that ties in what the patient has already said and helps them make a connection where they hadn't even realized how important a connection was waiting to be made. This is an example of where a practitioner can bring a little added awareness, along with other times when the practitioner can share important points of philosophy like *The Two Paths and the Compensation*. However, in any given case, it is best to leave it up to the Vis Dialogue to help reveal what is going on there. One is often surprised by what comes up! One case I had in the beginning of my practice was of an elderly woman in her 80s with myasthenia gravis. She told me that she developed myasthenia gravis following the passing of her husband. 'Clever' as I was at the time, I quickly concluded that this must be a case of grief – ailments from grief, as we call it in homeopathy. It couldn't have been further from the truth. Through Holistic Counseling, here is what was revealed in this woman's case (in a condensed form). Her husband died and she realized she had never loved him. Her next response to this was to feel extremely angry with herself for wasting her life with him. These thoughts then resulted in her feeling very guilty. The combination of guilt and anger turned toward herself made her body, the faithful puppy dog, also turn toward itself and she developed an auto-immune illness. I asked her if she thought this was serving her in any way. She said no. I then asked the big question, "Do you want to keep living this way?" She recognized that what had been occurring inside of her was a natural response, but she didn't want to keep doing it. She let herself off the hook and forgave herself for staying with him, and forgave her husband too for not being the man she had wanted to be with. I told her to bear with me that I was going to study her case and select a homeopathic remedy. It took me one week to finally suggest a remedy for her. I called her up and apologized for taking so long to get her the remedy, and she replied, "Oh it's just fine dearie. I don't need a remedy. All of my symptoms are gone."

Examples of Projecting and what NOT to do in Holistic Counseling practice – A patient comes with liver problems, so you immediately deduce that the cause of their illness is anger and you tell them this. Such a method of healing is working in the wrong direction. We must walk backward into the awareness of the cause by following the stream and observing, not projecting forward with knowing. Again, even if ultimately the practitioner is right in their assessment, it is the irreplaceable aha of helping a patient see for themselves that is far more valuable than them being told what the problem is. What we can say is that if someone has anger, it affects the liver. However, other things can affect the liver. Liver Qi stagnation can occur from suppressing sexual desire, and guilt can also affect the liver, which is a form of anger/judgment turned toward the self. The liver can also be affected by drinking alcohol chronically (to suppress emotions), and in many other ways. So to project on the person that has a problem with their liver by saying, "You have anger" is going backwards against The Healing Power of Nature.

Nature is a wonderful, beautiful thing that is fluid and lives in the quality of essence, rather than in any fixed or perfectly predictable fashion. This is where academic science goes wrong. It compartmentalizes the world too much by observing one slice of a phenomenon that is emitted by a much more fluid essence of Nature and holding the essence to that one slice.

True Holism and truly holistic practices and cosmologies deal with the whole essence of things. As in homeopathy, there are certain predictable patterns that can emerge from certain remedies. But in some cases, patterns emerged that have never been observed before and it is only through recognizing the essence in the totality of the symptoms, that one perceives the essence of the remedy as it lives in the pathology of that particular individual.

Another example of what NOT to do – A patient comes to visit you for help with knee problems. And you say, "*So, what are you not being flexible with in your life?*" Louise L. Hay's book, *You Can Heal Your Life*[14] is nice as an introduction. But don't consult it to determine the underlying cause of the illness with your patients. It was a ground-breaking book for its time, helping to establish a connection between mind and body, but it was just a baby step in understanding a much fuller picture of how patterns of illness originating in the mind can become manifest in the body. And the bigger picture is that it is not so well-defined. Only through individualized dialoguing, is the connection between mind and body made for a given patient.

During one of the first times of myself teaching Holistic Counseling, I had a beginner of the technique perform a demonstration in front of the class. The woman he was dialoguing with had a skin issue. Without even asking, "*How does the skin feel?*" and then following the answer up with more exploratory open-ended questions, this gentleman dove right in and asked, "*So what is getting under your skin?*" Where this could have been the ultimate discovery of the person (that there was in fact something "getting under her skin" emotionally), this is not an effective way of practicing the Vis Dialogue. To illustrate the difference between what to do and what not to do, there was a case of a woman who had pretty intense skin problems where nothing could help her. She finally did a Vis Dialogue. It took us a long time to get to the cause. I began by asking her how the skin felt. She said that it bothered her terribly. I asked how that felt. She said that it felt like it was crawling. I then asked, *"How does the crawling feel?"* She said, "Like something is under my skin." Aha! So that is good. She said, in her own words, "it feels like something was under my skin." Now, I could have looked for a parallel in her life, which is the technique of Holistic Counseling called *Reflecting Elsewhere*, wherein one asks, *"Is there anything or anywhere in your life that makes you feel this way?"* And I did, but she said, "No, not that I can think of." So then we explored areas of her life that were causing her difficulties. She said she had a lot of trouble with her daughter. Through various questions, she said her daughter was always on her mind. She said she bothers her so much, and then she said, spontaneously, "it's like my daughter is under my skin!" Within the instant of having said that, she had a strong intake of breath and a strong aha moment, recognizing that the very way in which the skin feels and the very language she used for both the skin and her daughter, established a mind-body connection and an understanding of what issue lay at the source of her skin problem. And this is often the case; that a person will use the same language, the same gestures, and it will feel the same between the symptoms of the body and the underlying cause in the mental-emotional sphere. She had some deep issues in her difficulty setting boundaries and saying no that she had to face within herself. So just snapping her fingers and making the skin problem go away in that moment was not possible, although the potential is always there for a person to be able to do so. She had to do some work in her relationship with her daughter and with herself, and she did, and the skin improved; a skin condition that she said she did everything to fix. All the drugs, the supplements – nothing would get rid of this itching, that, as we learned, was the result of an issue she had with her daughter, that had gotten under her skin. Interestingly, when I initially asked her if there was anywhere else in her life that she felt "was under her skin," she said no. There was not yet a bridge established where she could come to that awareness herself.

Chapter 25

Introduction to the Holistic Counseling Questions

I will begin by sharing an example case and how the questions proceed in a good dialogue, so that the reader can experience the questions in action, get a feel for what is involved, rather than just in a static and theoretical form. Discussion of the types of questions and when to use them will follow. There are areas of the case where I will also share valuable information about the practice from an "inside the head of the practitioner" perspective.

In the case, I indicate what my questions are by **bold italics**, and will share some thoughts in parentheses to comment on the case. In certain areas of the case, I have removed some of the responses that are not relevant for the progress of the case. It does create a slightly unrealistic accelerated account of the Vis Dialogue, but for the purpose of brevity and not to bore the reader with unnecessary reading, this is what I chose to do.

Case – 40-year-old woman with panics attacks and severe side effects from Ativan

Background of case: This case was of a woman who went on Ativan for anxiety and became extremely sick from it. She began having panic attacks and lost her appetite. She also became obsessive about her health and in particular, her caloric intake and specifically what foods she was eating (orthorexia). She lost a lot of weight and was unable to gain back her strength. She also had very low energy, was feeling depressed and hopeless. When I first began working with her, she seemed quite distraught and highly anxious. During our first appointment, she contacted some deep core issues from her past and she began to improve.

What follows is the third appointment working together, where she had a relapse of her anxiety, depression, and hopelessness.

"How are you feeling?"

"I am still tapering down on the medication. I've gotten down to about halfway – but it's doing a number on my endocrine system. I keep having these waves of being sick. Went and had my blood tested – my T3 is low. My thyroid is low. I am emotionally worried. My body seems to be so under. It is like I am shrinking away. I can see my ribs on both sides, and I just feel depleted.

It is overwhelmingly hopelessness.

Yesterday I went to see my naturopath. I went because I was concerned because I had stomach problems. Having extreme digestive problems – when I didn't have something that wasn't turned to mush. She thinks I have leaky gut. I also think my thyroid – it might be Hashimoto's. I don't have weight gain. I don't always have low thyroid – I sometimes have high thyroid. She thinks I should concentrate on healing my gut. I went to her because I didn't want the MD to push synthetic hormones on me."

(Here we see this naturopath works with the 'systems' model of medicine – so the idea is to heal the gut. As this case will later illustrate, this approach did nothing to address the underlying root of the problem of her condition which becomes clear as the questions proceed. In fact, because she already has a form of orthorexia (obsessed about all that she eats), the naturopath's prescription of the GAPS diet for the leaky gut actually made her anxiety worse, because it didn't address the root cause and it gave her even more to worry about in her food intake.

Many people, when they are very anxious about their health, will try to do everything they can in the mindset that, the more I do, the better it will be. It is just a means to compensate for their anxiety and their need for support (whatever their particular issue is in their "holistic" picture), because it is not an approach that normally works, and if it does, it will likely be suppressive over the patient's Vital Force and at the very least, confusing, to be led in so many different directions. When I see patients in a state like this, they often begin by telling me how they went to this doctor and that doctor, this naturopath, and this acupuncturist, etc. And this doctor said this and that doctor said that. And this doctor gave me this to take and that doctor gave me this and that to take. I ask them to just slow down, and to take a deep breath, and say, *"Ok, let's investigate what is really going on."* With a strong amplitude of anxiety like this patient had, it is easy to fall into it and panic and think, "What should I give this person to help them now?" rather than just asking the patient questions to zero in on the underlying problem.)

"Before this last wave – how were you doing?"

"I was doing a lot better. I felt I was doing better. I felt happier. I felt hopeful. I had some emotional breakthroughs and releases – let go of a lot of anger toward a lot of different people. Just felt generally more hopeful."

(This was hopeful and a sign that she was getting better, so now I had to investigate what went wrong? What sent things back off course?)

"Then what happened?"

"I began having some digestion problems and then... Also some kind of adrenal problems – I was having these episodes where the heart was squeezing, and then like an adrenaline rush. I had these before, but they were worse. But still, when it happens, it hits, and it makes me scared and makes me worried, and I just start losing hope."

"What does that feel like in your heart when it is happening?"

"I am afraid my heart is going to stop working and I am going to die."

"What if your heart stopped working and you died?"

"Who would take care of my kids? I would miss them, and

who would take care of them?

And I feel there is so much more I haven't experienced in this life…"

"What is it like taking care of your kids?"

(Note: At this point, I could have gone in other directions. I could have asked, *"What would happen if no one took care of you kids?"* Or, *"When do you experience this feeling the most?"* Or *"What else makes you feel this sort of worry and losing hope?"* There are often many paths that will lead to "Rome" i.e. the underlying cause. But I chose to ask this instead, about her children. The truth is, at many stages in the dialogue, a great many questions can be asked. The important thing is to ask a question that makes the patient move forward and deeper into their psyche. Some questions make a patient go backward, off on a tangent, or are irrelevant. One has to use their intuition and look for the signs of which aspects of a person to focus on. If I do ask a "dead-end" or irrelevant question, it's not a big problem at all. I will just say, *"Ok, let's go back a minute. When you said 'this', tell me about that,"* or something along those lines. Sometimes, when I ask a question, I feel a sense of loss of momentum in the answer, almost as if air is being deflated out of the conversation. I then switch my questioning to bring them more back in the direction that will lead deeper to the cause of their struggles and illness. With time, one begins to get a hang of the "right question" – which can mean any number of questions which leads the patient in the right direction – deeper down the "Rabbit Hole," and toward "Rome."

I also asked her, "What is it like taking care of your kids", because I have found that when a person fears death, the reason they fear death is intimately connected with the core of their underlying problem. One woman I was working with was so afraid to die that she didn't want to go to California to attend her son's wedding because she was afraid of an earthquake happening. When we explored her fear of death, what arose was

the feeling that if she dies, no one will see her. She will be invisible. This core feeling/belief just so happened to be permeating throughout her life. So death can often simply be an amplifier of the already-present fear and underlying core issue.)
So she answered:

"Feels overwhelming. Feels like I give a lot, and I don't get a lot back. It feels like a hopelessness."

"What is the connection there? How does the fact that you don't get back what you feel you give make you feel a hopelessness?"

"I feel like I am searching for love outside myself – so it is a codependent thing – so if I take care of these children and love them, then I will find the love I am seeking."

(This is actually a very, very insightful answer she expressed which comes from the fact that she is a person who works on herself, is self-aware, and also from our last two sessions together. Some people are very good at the Vis Dialogue i.e. using it to go deeper to answer questions to their problems. She is definitely an example of someone who is good at it – who can even jump into an awareness with fewer questions than I might need to ask someone else.)

"Where does this come from?"

"It's a pattern, a belief. I don't always recognize that is what I am doing. And now this pattern has come back to me. Giving love to kids, I am hoping I will get some validation/feedback."

"What makes you want to do this?"

"I have some false expectation that this is going to make me whole. I need to find it within myself. Presently, when I look inside myself, to find something to make me whole, I don't even know, who I am, or what I like to do, or what makes me happy. I just feel empty. There are people who get sick and give away all their possessions, and if I was going to die, what would I do? I don't even know. I just want to be in touch with myself, with my heart, and know myself and love myself. It just feels difficult to do that. I don't know why."

"What stands in the way of you knowing yourself?"

"It is negative thinking. Critical thoughts. A thought that loops – a negative loop. What's the use? I don't want to even try."

"Where does this negative thinking come from?"

"It's in my mother's voice. She has said stuff like that to me. I have held onto them – because it is what I have learned when I was younger."

"Do you want to keep holding onto them?"

"No!! I can let them go. Sometimes, it feels so overwhelming. It feels so large. She still speaks like that. I told my mom, I was halfway down off the medicine, and she just said, 'Ohhh, I thought you would be off of it by now.' I hardly ever get positive validation. I catch myself looking to her for validation – and I know it's not going to happen. A lot of times, she doesn't comment. But this time, she said that, and it hit the little girl in me, I let her words discourage me."

(So here we see the beginning of a thread. She looks to her mother for validation and this is what she looks for from her children as well. So we see the same issue reflected over two situations. That is a thread. That shows us we're on the right path. Also, the fear of death brings up the feeling of "who will care for my children?" and this brings up two of the principles and metaphors of Holistic practice. The first is that she uses loving and taking care of her children as a compensation for her core issue of not feeling validated. Secondly, there is a *natural-healthy response mingled with an added unhealthy-element* here. It's natural and healthy to want to take care of your kids and it is unhealthy to mingle one's own need to compensate for one's issue into the mix of taking care of the children.)

"When did you have this conversation in relation to you having this new wave of low energy, digestive issues and depression return?"

"It started right after this conversation with my mother."

(Bingo! So there it is – the trigger that made her go from doing well to having a relapse. It is therefore most significant and related to the root cause of her problems.)

"I was happy. I was doing well. We've had a really long winter, and I hadn't spoken to her and kept my distance and was doing well. I had to call her and ask for help with money. There was no way we could have had it down without her help. So I have had to talk to her, recently. I fall into those old patterns, the more I need to have communication with her, or contact. I feel it is hard to keep my boundaries. When I get around her, I let my aura down and I let her in."

"To do what?"

"When I am feeling well – I can keep my boundaries up. But when I feel vulnerable –I ask for help and for love. And I remember going outside, and feeling like a little girl, like a victim, crying, not knowing what to do. My boyfriend isn't 'fixy techy.' He doesn't know how. So I had to call her –I was feeling like a victim and vulnerable, and I didn't mentally prepare myself to have those boundaries up. I have done that all my life – looking to her for the love that I am not going to get from her. I really thought I had accepted it. I have had this conversation lots of times and journalled about it. So I didn't realize I was back to that point. I really think it has something to do with this house, because my stepfather and her bought it for me and gave it to me, but it kind of feels there are strings attached. A way for her to keep a hold or finger on me, and control me. That is what it feels like. I don't want to live here anymore. I want to live somewhere else. I just... I don't know how it will be possible right now. I didn't even realize when they gave it to me, it is not even in my name."

"You said, looking to her for help – you went into a little girl and victim state?"

"I think it is just surrounding the house. With other things, I don't feel that way.

With help with my kids – I can ask others... With my mother, it was a major thing."

"What makes it so large with your mother?"

"Most of my life, I have allowed this codependent thing to go on, where my mom, she doesn't give what I need emotionally, she gives financially. I keep myself in this "poverty" – situations where I am going to need her help. I go back to that spot inside where I have to call mom for help."

(At this point, another really important part of the thread begins to reveal itself inside the tapestry of her life. She feels her mother doesn't give her emotional love. She just gives financial love. With her children, she feels like she doesn't receive what she needs, and just gives more. She also feels like she is trying to give to them in an effort to get the love she feels she needs. Also, the house is a financial attachment to her mother, who she feels, uses the financial element to control her and keep her "dependent." This is a vicious cycle for her.)

"There have been times when I don't fall back into that. Something tied with the age of my daughter and my age? She is four now, and when I was four, it locked something in. Feels like when I was four, something changed for me... It just feels like, in my heart, some attachment I put into my heart."

"What is it that you put there?"

"I put my worth there, in my heart. It's where Divine love, self-love comes from. I can access that in my heart. But there is something else there that I put there, that I don't know how to describe. That is where I put... that is what love was... so that is where I stuck these beliefs. I put them in my heart, because that is what I thought love was."

(This was another major awareness. She is realizing that she puts the limiting beliefs that came from her mother into her heart because she thought that was love. That's really important.)

"Do you want to continue to put that in your heart?"

"No!"

"Is it ok to let it go from your heart?"

"Yes."

"Can you sense it is leaving and that it doesn't have to dwell anymore?"

"There is a part that is fighting it. I don't know why. It feels like my ego. My ego has been so used to thinking this was truth, it is scared of change."

(This is not uncommon in cases – to resist letting go out of fear of change. In her case, in the end, it didn't affect her too much. But in other cases, I describe what to do with this fear of change in Chapter 32 on *What to do When the Case is Not Advancing or is Stuck*.)

She continues:

"If I let this go, how am I going to live? How am I going to know myself?"

I then say:

"Let me summarize until this point. All the thoughts cluttered in your heart that you have adopted from your mother have stood in the way of knowing yourself and knowing your value and who you really are, because the thoughts you stored there, in your heart, which you thought was love, have remained blocking you from knowing yourself."

(whenever I give feedback, I ask something like, *"Does that resonate with you? Is that accurate?"*)

"Does that sound about right?"

"Yes. When you say it, it is so eloquent, and I know, later on, when I try to tap into it, and I want to reassure myself, the thoughts will be gone... I continue to put myself into those situations.

Sometimes, it's hard to slow down and notice I am doing it, until I get to the point where I am depleting myself."

"What is it that you tend to do that you don't always notice?"

"Her not validating that I was doing well coming off the

drugs. When I am looking outside for validation, I am affirming I have no worth. I don't want to affirm that anymore. I am feeling an ache in my heart right now, it hurts... I've tried to be more spiritual lately, and just ask for Divine Intuition... show me. But I felt so overwhelmed."

"How do you feel inside right now?"

(I asked her this because she became very frantic and sped up. I could sense she was reconnecting with herself, which, as she mentioned earlier, is at the heart of her problem, being disconnected. Having her check in to how she was feeling was a good way for her to connect with her heart. This is a technique in Holistic Counseling that can always be used to calm a situation down or to get a patient to reconnect with themselves when they're off too deeply into the intellect and disconnected from their feelings. She is saying it hurts. So I knew at this point in the dialogue this was the direction she needed to go. The fact that she is speaking about these issues and feeling them, this is already moving in the right direction. What comes next confirms that. Remember, she was trying many things in a desperate attempt to feel better and nothing was helping.)

She answers:

"I don't feel as hopeless. I still have the ache in my heart. It is just an ache. I have had it there for a while. Through this whole dialogue process. It feels like a hurt. I have let myself be hurt. It feels sore. It feels like a bruise."

"What has made you be hurt?"

"It is because I let myself be hurt by looking for validation where I know I am not going to get it. Like a sabotage. My heart is saying, the love you need is right here, why are you looking outside and letting all of these other emotions and other things affect you, when it is right here?!?! My heart is trying to talk to me."

(This is a big statement for her, as she just finished saying she doesn't know herself because her heart is filled with ideas that came from her mother that she thought were love. It is difficult to detect this just from the words on the page, but the emotion of the room went from feeling frantic and her voice being tight and tense, to opening up, calming down, and her voice really reflecting the inner depth she was contacting. It is also a good sign when the patient says something like what she said – that she cannot know herself, and now, she is saying something that indicates otherwise.)

"I still feel this fear there, in my heart."

"What is the fear about?"

"I have this fear that if I let go of the pain and the thoughts from my mother that my heart will stop also. My worth is so tied up into this, what I have carried. I am afraid that my heart just might be empty."

"Can you take a guess about what is in your heart?"

(This was a bit of a strange question to ask and a bit of a jump here and not so fluid as asking the next question in the stream of questions and answers. Another question could have been, *"And what if your heart is empty?"* Or *"How is your worth so tied up into all of this?"* but instead, I asked, *"Can you take a guess about what is in your heart?"* because I really wanted to just keep her focused on her heart. That seemed to be the most important place for her to keep exploring and it ended up working just fine and she came up with some very amazing answers.)

"It feels like going back to the essence of me, from birth. It just feels like really old… that is what is there, at the bottom of it. It feels like I have to go all the way back, all the way back and start back over. I don't know why this makes me sad. It feels like going way back even before birth, and starting over."

(At this point, she is almost in a trance-like state, where she is getting many answers that are coming right up from her very essence.)

"Right in this moment, feel like it is happening, like being

back in the womb. What do you sense there?"

"My soul in the womb felt regret for choosing my mother. Once I got in there, it was like, 'Oh shit, who is this woman? What did I just do?!?!'"

"What did you do then?"

"I immediately started doing the co-dependent thing. Feeling like I had to take on her fear. She had fear from the moment she got pregnant and all of her negative thinking, and the situation with my dad wasn't favorable, so I began taking it all on... from the womb."

"Can you change what you did then, now?"

"Yes!! Yes!! I feel lighter... I feel lighter." (She was weeping deeply at this point. Releasing a lot.)

"My soul feels lighter.

I still have the pain there, but my soul... I actually feel some hope."

(I let her rest in this place for a moment and then asked:)

"Can you accept your choice in the mother you chose?"

"Yes! Because I wouldn't be who I am without her, if I hadn't made that choice. It took me 40 years and now I have the chance to open up!"

There was some celebrating and light discussion about her awareness and all the far reaching implications for her life. And here we ended the dialogue.

This was truly a big breakthrough for her. I then suggested she go and journal all the implications for opening her heart and letting go of the codependent attachment to her mother's beliefs and fears and unhappiness. All of this was related to her digestive issues and her gut problems, which were closely connected to her anxiety. It helped her a lot.

Another interesting aspect of this case was that she had some pretty intense physical issues going on. She had lost so much weight following the health problems that resulted from the Ativan that her ribs were showing. At one point, she had developed jaundice. This made her anxiety and panic attacks worse. One doctor actually told her that when you have jaundice, there's a good chance you're going to die. I did some research and discovered that jaundice is a well-known side effect of the Ativan. None of her doctors had told her this. And what is more important is that she went on the Ativan in the first place to suppress the anxiety she was feeling, which was all part of the dynamic she had grown up with doing so many things to get validated, because she didn't feel validated by her mother, instead she allowed all of her mother's fears and issues to come into her heart (following her sense of disappointment in her mother being the way she was), which blocked her from her own sense of self. So she was searching to be validated and to find who she was and the lack of that connection to herself and her need to be validated made her feel a great sense of anxiety and overwhelm (because, as she discovered herself – My heart is saying, the love you need is right here, why are you looking outside and letting all of these other emotions and other things affect you, when it is right here?!?!) She used Ativan to try to "fix" that anxiety – that worsened the underlying Vital Force mistunement and sent her into a spiral of very bad health issues which forced her to explore her life and herself. Now, what is interesting is that I believe the negative effects of the Ativan would continue until she resolved the underlying reason behind why she went on the Ativan in the first place. This is also the phenomenon in healing that I shared in the previous chapter regarding chronic injuries that are not getting better.

Chapter 26

The Actual Holistic Counseling Questions

As I have mentioned, and as you saw in the first case example, The Vis Dialogue is based mostly on non-directive questions. There are some instances where directive questions work fine, without interfering with the patient's own process, but for the most part, the spelt bread and organic butter of the Holistic Counseling Vis Dialogue is comprised of non-directive questions. And there is a good reason for that. Non-directive questions allow for the answer to arise from within the patient. This permits a process of getting to the core to occur in the most accurate and unbiased fashion. Directive questions have more of the input of the practitioner woven into them and imply that the practitioner sees the answer and so should the patient. This invariably begins to throw off the smooth and harmonious-with-Nature unfolding of a case when it is done too much. Every practitioner should endeavor to use mostly non-directive questions as they are the way to help set people free from their suffering. Using directive questions is, however, not a sin, and with experience, it may become clear when a little directive question can have a positive impact. I'll discuss further where using directive questions is helpful.

Non-Directive Questions

Definition from Merriam-webster.com:

"Non-directive: of, relating to, or being psychotherapy, counseling, or interviewing in which the counselor refrains from interpretation or explanation but encourages the client (as by repeating phrases) to talk freely."[15]

That is the main idea of Holistic Counseling. To ask a question which is non-directive that holds no suggestion or projection of what the right answer is.

"How do you feel about that?"

"What makes you think that?"

"Where does that come from?"

I noticed when I work with some people, they do not respond well to intellectual questions, whereas others do. Usually someone who doesn't respond well to intellectual-type questions will do better with emotional-type questions and vice versa. *"What makes you think that?"* is more of an intellectual-type question and *"How does that make you feel?"* is more of an emotional-type question. When asking non-directive questions, keeping a balance between intellectual and emotional questions is a good idea, so you can elicit responses from both the intellectual realm and emotional realm. However, in some cases, if a person is largely more emotional or intellectual, asking the kinds of questions specific for their "type" will yield more results. In time, a person who is very intellectual can learn to get in touch with their feelings and will be able to respond to emotional-type questions, especially if they have blocked their feelings due to certain beliefs about their feelings, e.g. "My mother was too emotional, and she was so weak. I told myself I would never be like that." Working with someone who comes from such a background can help them let go of the control they believe they need by avoiding their emotions, and can help them get into a more balanced state. Conversely, where someone has grown up doubting their intellectual capacities and feels more comfortable in an emotional state of being, they will at first respond better to emotional-type questions, because intellectual-type questions can trigger the very doubt in their own intelligence that makes them stay away from the intellectual side of things. In time, they can recognize their own doubt in themselves and the beliefs they have adopted to diminish their intellectual side, and can respond to more intellectual-type questions which will help them get even further down the Rabbit Hole into the core of their limiting belief systems. In the end, a balanced person is always a better version of themselves than a very one-sided person.

Examples of Non-Directive Questions (and type):

"What makes you feel that way?" (emotional)

"What do you mean by that?" (intellectual)

"How does that feel?" (emotional)

"Where do you think you got that idea?" (intellectual)

"How long have you felt that way?/When did it start?" (emotional)

"What makes you think that.... is true?" (intellectual)

"Tell me more." (neutral)

"I don't understand what you mean by that?" (intellectual)

There is one question-word that is not present in this list, and you may have noticed, I did not use it in the first example case. That question-word is the word, "Why?" Why do we not use the question-word why?

There are a few reasons for this. The main reason is through experience. It is much more difficult for people to try to answer a *"Why do you think that is?"* question than a *"What makes you think that?"*

"What *makes you think that?"* requires a person to focus in on a specific answer, which is like keeping them focused on the path of breadcrumbs through their mind. *"Why do you think that is?"* invites people to speculate and to theorize and does not usually yield a concise answer. For this reason, I do not ever ask people questions using the word "Why?" It doesn't take long to convert one's habit from *"why do you?"* to *"what makes you?"* Lou Klein, the great homeopath, also does not use the word "why?" when questioning his patients. I originally got the idea of not using the word "Why?" in my Holistic Counseling practice from Lou.

There is a well-developed list of more specialized questions later, along with different questions and techniques one can employ the use of for certain key situations in practice. Knowing these specialized questions and techniques and where to specifically apply them is very helpful in practice.

Directive Questions

"Are you aware of what you are saying by that?"
"Is it possible that you may not want to face this?"
"Are you projecting in this instance?"
"Do you have a difficulty around men? Women? Authority?"
"Do you have an issue with your mother? Father? With your sexuality?"

Those questions are directive. Can you sense the difference? And can you imagine the different impact it has on the dialogue? There are ways of being even more directive, where you are giving a piece of advice woven into the question.

For example:

"Wouldn't it be better if you just walked away?" or
"Can you see how this is a futile cause for you?"

There are some directive questions that are better than others. These questions are almost not questions at all, but rather, statements of advice from the practitioner, disguised as questions. It is important for the practitioner not to fool themselves into thinking they are asking questions when they are really just giving advice in question form. This sort of counseling completely changes the dynamic from the patient knowing what is true for themselves to the doctor thinking that they know what is true/right for the patient.

I have found that the time to ask the directive questions is when we have already established an awareness of what a person's belief is and where a person's problem lies. This may occur during the dialogue and often happens toward the end of the session, where, once the problems are out in the open, the directive questions can then be used to help a patient focus in on something which will assist them to focus in a particular direction that will be helpful for them.

For example, in one case of a woman in her seventies with myasthenia gravis, after many of the standard, open-ended questions were asked, the patient got to this point, which I had her summarize for herself:

"I deny myself, and I allow others to tell me who I am, in order to be loved by them because I fear they will withdraw from me and leave me alone as an outsider if I am strong within myself."

Then I asked a directive question:

"Where is your mistake in that situation?"

This serves the purpose to get the patient to recognize and then express their mistake, i.e. their choice in the matter. (Asking this sort of a question is done gently and with a lot of compassion. Patients then can understand it that way and in no way feel condemned by such a question.)

She responded:

"I think there are three mistakes. To allow others to tell me who I am. And to think that they will love me if they can tell me who I am. It is easier to deny myself, than to fight/battle for myself."

A few questions could then be asked:

"What makes it easier for you to deny yourself, than to fight/battle for yourself?"

Once that is explored, we can bring back the patient to remember the mistakes that are inherent in their bottom line beliefs and responses to their life. And ask the life-changing question: *"Do you want to keep living that way?"* (that is, in and of itself, a directive question.)

Another directional question which is appropriate once a person states the errors in innocence that they made, in their life that was not good for them?

"Can you forgive yourself and accept yourself for those things happening?"

In her particular case, she said "Yes. Yes, I can!"

In a way, directional questions can be used to get the patient to state they are in fact going to make those changes in their lives.

In the case of the woman with body dysmorphic disorder, through the dialogue process, she discovered that her mother played a strong role in her life, in the sense that her mother controlled, denied, judged, or was generally the main perpetrator of the wound; we can then ask a directive question:

"What were some of the messages coming from your mother relating to your body?"

The idea here is again that once an awareness is established, the directive question can then help to connect the dots for the patient. It can be like a form of feedback, yet leaving it open for the patient to make the connection themselves.

Another example of a directive question we can ask when the person has already responded to whether they wish to keep living this way or not. When they say no, the next question is as follows:

"What if you do look at your body, from time to time, the way you used to? What are you going to do about that?"

This directive question is to isolate a specific situation to help the person anticipate and to plan. Hopefully, their response is, "I will just remind myself of what I have learned here today." It is ok for the practitioner to explain, at this stage, that it is normal that they may slip back into the old pattern, but just to encourage them in the awareness that they have made and the new choices they are making to heal themselves.

Even when asking directive questions, it is important for us to remain non-directive energetically. Imagine how it feels when you really need to have someone see it your way. That is an energetic pull. Do not pull or push on the patient energetically when asking any type of question, expecting them to see the answer that you see, or think you see. This is another way in which most beginners struggle. It is hard to let go and allow the person to come up with answers themselves, partly because, when one is being the practitioner, it is easy to feel that they are in the driver's seat, and in that position, one has authority and power. That idea comes mostly from our old model of medicine that is becoming antiquated – the idea that the doctor is responsible for the patient's health. Working with someone in a vulnerable position also quickly and easily calls into the foreground the practitioner's sense of self-worth and their own personal power. If a practitioner's self-worth or feeling of personal power is shaky, he/she will more easily fall into wanting to provide advice and into asking more directive questions. The incorrect thinking, which is highly alluring, is to go straight into believing that, "They are vulnerable and suffering. They need me to help. I will show them the way!" It can be quite a drug for the practitioner, an alluring balm of importance of power. The practitioner must avoid this as much as possible, as it can actually be harmful for a patient if the practitioner is wrong in their perception. Even if they are right, as I have mentioned, it creates an unhealthy dynamic where the patient needs the answers from the practitioner. This is very important because it is quite common for people with many issues themselves to go into practicing counseling/psychotherapy. "We go into what we need!" There, they have a platform to be important, to have answers for people, often counterbalancing their own feelings of inadequacy and powerlessness in themselves. These sorts of practitioners create needy, codependent relationships with their patients, and they should really be in counseling themselves. Our goal is to become obsolete, not to get patients dependent on our insights and advice. Ultimately, we all have our own insecurities, and everyone likes to be in a position where they can help others. So initially, when a practitioner begins practicing the way of Holistic Counseling, it is best to get it right from the start and not to be steering, pulling, pushing, or forcing views on people, even if it is hard in the beginning to let go of that control and even if it is only on the energetic or intentional level. The truth is, that by letting go of the external control in one's practice, one is ultimately disconnecting from their need to get power and self-esteem from the outside. One is also affirming the truth that the answers to our most pressing and important questions live within ourselves; by helping another see that we also get in the habit and have an impact on ourselves for the very same. *As we do unto others, so are we actually doing unto ourselves.*

Even if a practitioner doesn't have many of their own issues in their practice, many of the models of counseling and psychotherapy involves the practitioner telling the patient what their problem is, because they have gone to school and have a diploma and are a kind of authority on what is right and wrong in a person's thinking. Also, sitting in the practitioner's seat, it is often quite easy to see what a person's problem is, especially after some time when the thread is established. It is then most tempting to push a patient into seeing what their problem is. Many practitioners get to this point and they get a little frustrated because the patient is so close to seeing it! Pushing a patient, asking too many directive questions with the intention of knowing the answer is not nearly as effective as trusting in the patient and in The Healing Power of Nature, and it is why our patients have asserted that one session of Holistic Counseling was like years of therapy. And many have said, they have never been asked such questions and gotten to such a deep under-standing of themselves in such a short amount of time.

What happens when we use too many directive questions?

I can tell you what happens to me. I get a very bad feeling inside of myself. It's like my gut knows I am violating some important universal principle even before I became fully aware of what I was doing. It's also because of a subtle dynamic that occurs between patient and doctor when this occurs. When we ask too many directive questions, normally it is because we feel we have the answers, or we should be in control. Most of the time, the intention, as nice as it is, is to help the person. However, the desire to help someone along with the control and directiveness is a formula for potential disaster, because it is an invitation for the person's unhealthy, blocked, and negative energy to be transferred right into the practitioner.

When I went wrong in this way in my practice, I have been honest enough with myself to watch this dynamic happening. I began getting frustrated with the patient's lack of seeing the answers that I was seeing, or that I thought I was seeing. I, of course, wanted to help them, and so I began throwing in my awareness into my questions, creating the "perfect" directive questions for the patient to see the light. What then happens is that the ego or the part of their illness that is invested in being sick and attached to their illness begins to push back. I am pushing, so why shouldn't they push back? This almost never fails. What results is a tug of war between the patient and the doctor which is the very last thing either party desires in the dialogue. That is one of my least favorite feelings. It is so contrasting to the kind of peace and joy that result from being detached enough and trusting enough to allow the patient to come up with the answers on their own, at their own pace, even if it takes longer than I would like it to. Since I hit this wall and experienced this tug of war on several occasions, I have really committed to avoid it at all costs, mostly for the fact that it doesn't work. Later, with more experience, I have grown into the trust in knowing that the answer really and truly must come from the patient. I suppose at some point I shifted from that being a concept I told myself because I believed it to be correct, to a concept that I had no doubt in as I experienced the truth of it emanating from The Healing Power of Nature. And so now, when I encounter a patient that is not going deeper, I know that with time, and enough questions, they will get where they need to go, so there is no point in diving into directive/controlling mode.

As an aside, I'd like to bring about some balance to this last awareness of trusting the answer to come from the patient, which is totally and completely true unto itself. It doesn't mean, however, that the practitioner cannot put a little pressure on the patient to get them to answer questions they don't feel comfortable with. This is because the illness has a way of wanting to survive. And a person's sick side can be more in control than their own true and healthy self. And what is a practitioner there to serve – the sick side of a person, or the healthy side? A practitioner must therefore recognize when a patient is acting out of their illness and continue to ask the difficult questions to work toward a breakthrough and not let someone off the hook too easily when the going gets tough. Sure, if someone says, with full conviction, "I really must stop. I really cannot go on any further," then I stop. Otherwise, I press on, *gently (female)* and *firmly (male)*, with the non-directive questions, getting them ever closer to the release of the part of them that is in resistance to health.

In summary, non-directive questions are the grass-fed, free-range meat and organic potatoes of the Holistic Counseling Vis Dialogue, and it is especially important to not use directive questions out of frustration that the case is not advancing or opening up. Directive questions are used at certain key spots, mostly toward the end of the Vis Dialogue to focus in on the choice and get a patient to unchoose their core belief, but also where the truth has already been revealed by the patient and the practitioner is asking something to help them make a connection or make a plan with that already revealed truth. In the example cases that follow, I will demonstrate where I have used directive questions and what made it ok in that instance. And sometimes, it is simply for the fact that you cannot think of a non-directive question that you can ask a directive question. The idea is to keep the flow going. Some practitioners have reported that they were really struggling at a certain point in the dialogue and one or two directive questions really helped the case open up and advance. That's the idea. And remember, it's not a sin to ask directive questions.

Let's continue with more of the Vis Dialogue main principals.

Go Into and Through the Negative and the Fear

Just as facing one's fears brings about the most healing, going through a person's negative thinking patterns and thoughts will be the most healing and liberating for them. So, another one of the important principles of the Vis Dialogue is to *go into and through the negative and the fear*. It means where there is pain, fear, judgment, struggle, and suffering, ask a question to explore that, to go into it. This is very homeopathic in nature. Whenever a person's fear is revealed in practice, the plan is to go into and through it by asking the next question about it. For example, a patient says "I don't like when people look at me."

So the next question, to go into and through the negative, would be,

"What is it about people looking at you that you don't like?"

Or it can simply be:

"Tell me about what you don't like about people looking at you."

This begins the process of opening up the negativity and fear, to get to the bottom of it and begin unravelling it by revealing the underlying choice that is the source of the charge behind the negativity and fear.

As another example, a patient states:

"If I make a mistake, people will think I am stupid."

So naturally here, to go into and through the negative, we would ask,

"And what if people think you are stupid?"

Their next answer can reveal any number of thoughts or issues that would then be explored by following the stream with another open-ended, non-directive question, and also by applying the principle of going into and through the negative.

Vis Dialogue Summary Until Now: So for now, in our understanding of the Holistic Counseling Dialogue, we have: **Ask non-directive questions, reserve directive questions for key points in the Dialogue, and remember the important principle of going into and through the negative.**
These principles, and the next few that will follow, are simple, but they work. As I have observed beginners in Holistic Counseling, I notice that they understand these principles but do not necessarily apply them in their selection of questions to use. It is important that they are applied, because they yield the best and most healing results.

Next principle.

Follow the Stream. Ask Questions by Going with the Flow.

Now that we have looked at the type of questions, the question is, when do we ask questions and how do we ask questions?

The basic idea is to allow a person to continue to express themselves until they are no longer speaking, or they are no longer expressing anything that is helping them get deeper towards an understanding of themselves. One then selects the next question that emerges from what they just previously said.

For example, if someone says, "I really don't like speaking in front of more than one person." The easiest way of asking a question about that is to take exactly what they have said and to ask the very next question that presents itself. *"What makes you not like speaking in front of more than one person?"*

Or if someone says, "I really feel small around educated people." The next question would be, *"What makes you feel small around educated people?"* Or one could ask, *"What is it about educated people that makes you feel small?"* The question is subtly different but can yield quite a different response. Either way would be fine.

There are many permutations of the questions that can be asked, and a practitioner can be really flexible with them. I have come to learn that the expression of "All paths lead to Rome," is very appropriate for asking Holistic Counseling questions. A patient has a problem. As you begin to ask them questions, you will hit a vein of energy inside of them that is connected to their core issues and wound. This leads to "Rome" – the main underlying issue. So where one finds the vein, or the thread, and one follows it, there is no wrong question there. This takes the pressure off us practitioners to know we will get there eventually, by keeping on with the questions.

A 'poor' question or a question of little use would be one which gets off the vein or path leading to Rome and leads nowhere. A practitioner would experience this as having momentum and then sensing that they are not getting anywhere.

I like the metaphor of rock climbing when looking for questions to ask. In rock climbing, we seek footholds and handholds to grab onto so we can climb higher. Some climbs are harder than others, and only a few difficult handholds will be available to climb a mountain. Some climbs are easier and there are many large handholds and footholds to climb with. When a person shows a great deal of emotion surrounding a subject, that subject becomes an easy foothold/handhold to begin exploring. When a person is very shut down and "not giving anything away", the footholds and handholds are harder to find. But with the right patience, and at times, with some intuition, we can find those difficult footholds/handholds. One takes the next step by following the next foothold/handhold that emerges following the previous question. In this way, we go with the flow. One can use the metaphor of climbing the mountain, but I also love the metaphor from *Alice in Wonderland* where one is exploring "the Rabbit Hole." This is more appropriate because we really are descending into the subconscious mind of our patients as we ask questions that get us deeper and deeper. I will even say to the patient, *"We are going to see how far down into the Rabbit Hole this issues goes."* And in so doing, we can still look for those footholds and handholds which allow us to descend gently and in a stepwise fashion. It is through the negative that we find handholds and footholds to explore in the Rabbit Hole.

Keep to the Context of the Stream

When asking questions, it is best to ask a question that sticks to the general context of what was last said or revealed by the patient. When you begin exploring with a patient by following the stream and going with the flow, there should be a continuity between what the patient says and the next question you ask. There is a question and an answer that is related to the question. This is keeping to the context of the stream. For example, someone says ,"I get so confused when I am faced with challenges."

A good question that follows the stream and keeps to the context would be, *"What is it about challenges that makes you confused?"* Or we can also ask, *"Tell me about the confusion?"* Or, *"What sort of challenge would make you confused?"* These are all questions that follow the stream and keep to the context of the last thing spoken by the patient. Examples of questions that *do not* keep to the same context would be, *"How does that feel?"* That doesn't make sense with what the patient is saying. Or, *"What makes you think that?"* That is also out of context and not the time to ask that question. It will confuse a patient because they are stating that they do, in fact, get confused when faced with challenges. So if you were to ask, *"What makes you think that?"* The patient will say, "Because I do." It's not a good question because it's out of context. It's not the end of the world to ask out of context questions, but each question is best selected to be most appropriate based on the stream and matching the context.

Another example, a patient just states, "I am always trying so hard to prove to people that I am competent."

Good questions keeping with flow of stream and context: *"What makes you try so hard to prove that you're competent?"* Or, *"What is it like for you to always be trying to prove you're competent?"* Or, *"What does being competent get you?"* Or, *"What if you're not competent?"*

Questions that are *not* in keeping with the context: *"How does that feel?"* Or, *"What makes you think that?"* Or, *"What is so hard about trying?"*

So keeping to the context is an important principle of the Vis Dialogue.

Sometimes, however, you will find yourself exploring a train of thought with a patient that will change into what seems like a new direction, and may seem unrelated to the previous line of questioning. Open ended, non-directive questions that get a patient to reflect inwardly, deeply, have a way of evoking old, buried memories. Sometimes, the memories that get triggered are really what the issue is all about. It's like you're exploring a forest and you wake up a bear sleeping in a nearby cave. You didn't realize you were going to do so. You thought you were just exploring the forest. But lo and behold! Out comes a bear! So if you do hit a pocket of memory which was close, but not quite on the track of the direction of questions you'd been asking, don't worry about it. Follow the new course, the new stream that emerges. It will take you down the Rabbit Hole even deeper and toward the core issue.

A practitioner can also develop their own favorite questions, and favorite ways of asking questions. I sometimes even just say *"Really?"* in response to someone's previous statement, as a way of getting them to continue to explain themselves further. The idea is to get them to go with the flow. The understanding is that with time, and via this method of non-directive, open ended, non-judgmental questions, a person *does* and *will* get deeper into contact with themselves, so just keep them answering the next, and often, deeper question. I write this also because beginner practitioners often say that they don't know what to ask next. I suggest printing out the list of questions, or memorizing the list, so that one has, at their fingertips, an array of questions that they could ask. And then, in the moment, it is just a matter of asking the question that seems to best suit the situation.

A portion of a case example that employs the principals we've learned up until now:

"The other day, I was so angry. I felt angry all day."

"What were you angry about?"

"I was so mad at my neighbor for making so much noise."

"What was it about your neighbor making so much noise that made you so angry?"

"I felt so angry because they weren't being very respectful of me and my space."

"How did it feel when they weren't being respectful?"

"I felt disregarded, ignored, like I didn't matter. Only they mattered."

"How does it make you feel when someone behaves as if only they matter and you don't matter, or like they ignore you?"

"Very, very angry."

"What is about that that makes you angry?"

"It's because they are so selfish. All they care about is themselves."

"And what if someone cares only about themselves?"

"It's like they don't acknowledge your existence."

"What is it like to not have your existence acknowledged?"

"It's very painful."

What does the pain feel like?

"It feels like being left alone."

"What is being left alone like for you?"

"It's like there is nobody there who cares about you."

What is that like for you?

"It is like nobody loves me."

Now at this point, we would continue to then try to find a parallel for when this started. The question to do so could be, *"Is there anywhere else in your life that made you feel this way?"* (this is what I call a *"Reflecting Elsewhere"* Question.) These help a person see that the very fundamental idea or wound that they carry came from somewhere outside of them, either from an experience, or from the ideas or ways of being of another person. Therefore, it is not something carved in stone, and not something they have to continue to live, as if it is the ultimate capitol T truth that they are doomed to live by. This is very helpful. What is also already immediately helpful is that the person can become more detached about the experience that they think was really upsetting them – regarding the neighbor being very loud and disrespectful. They are not ultimately that emotionally angry about the neighbor playing music. It is that it makes them feel the way they did as a child, when they felt unloved. This pain they carry is being triggered by the neighbor, so they project onto the neighbor their anger. When the underlying issue is removed, the outer world can actually spontaneously change, i.e. the neighbor gets this flash of insight that maybe not everyone in the world around wants to listen to their music. Or, they are also in a much lighter place to go up and say, "Hey my man, do you mind turning down your music a little? It's a bit loud for me over here." Why not, eh? And if that doesn't help change the environment, the emotional charge surrounding the situation is discharged and the person either pays it less mind, or finds a more harmonious environment to be in. When old wounds are continuously dragged up from being in a certain situation, it can be difficult to leave that situation. It's like we are locked in a battle with it, as it resonates with the past, we are attracted to it to try to resolve our wounds. Once we let go and release the past, we no longer need to stay in that same situation any longer and are free to move on, or the Universe "senses" our release and the situation outside changes naturally.

Here is something *not to do* in practice: Don't try to "soften" a directive question that you want them to have an answer for by being vague and indirect, thinking this makes it non-directive. Sometimes, we can see the answer. It's true. We really can. But how to get them to see it? What I have learned *not to do* is to throw in a directive question where I have a specific answer in mind that I want them to see and I try to "disguise it" as a non-directive question. Patients get completely confused and it never, ever works.

For example, I can see that the patient is very logical and they judge when people are emotional and that is why they are judging their very own emotions. So here is what I asked. *"Is there somewhere else in your life that you judge that is like how you feel inside of yourself about your emotions?"* (How confusing is that?!?!)

Once I do that, I might as well come right out and tell them: *"You judge your own emotions because you judge emotions in others."* It could of course be the opposite as well, but the dialogue in this particular case unfolded such that they became aware that they judge emotions in others before they recognized that they are doing it in themselves, and that is what was causing the most health issues for them now.

I have caught myself doing this sometimes and it always makes patients stumble and not know what to answer. Most of the time, they will say, "Uhhh, sorry. I don't understand what you're asking me." Even with patients who are really excellent at responding to my non-directive questions, doing this sort of thing never yields an answer. It has so much to do with intention. Since my intention is directive and *as if I have the answer already* (or I *think* I have the answer), it's like the patient blanks out. I have the answer so how are they supposed to know the answer themselves? That "doctor knows all" dynamic can easily fall into place. It also throws a wrench in the works after asking so many wonderful non-directive questions that it stops up the brain. The patient cannot answer. And they shouldn't be able to. I might as well either come right out and say it, give feedback where I then add extra information, or ask the question more directly. *"Can you see that you have a hard time accepting emotions inside of yourself because you also judge it in others?"* I have confused them with that previous sort of a mixed up, half-non-directive, half-directive question. Even if they don't know that I am not supposed to ask such directive questions during the Vis Dialogue, you can see the direct evidence of this kind of a mixed-up question when you do it. I apologize immediately when I try to do this and I say, *"Sorry, that wasn't a very good question."* Because it wasn't. We have a laugh about it and then I select a better question for the moment.

Vis Dialogue Summary Until Now: So for now, in our understanding of the Holistic Counseling Dialogue, we have: **Ask non-directive questions, remember the important principle of going into and through the negative, go with the flow by asking the next question that naturally presents itself from the last thing the person said, keep to the context of the flow, and reserve directive questions for key points in the Dialogue.**

What I will share next is how to use feedback in the Vis Dialogue.

Chapter 27

Feedback – The Different Methods of Feedback

Feedback is the technique of repeating back to a patient what they have already said. It serves to establish trust. "Hey, this person is actually listening to what I have to say." It also helps a person recall what they have said, and can bring a deeper light of understanding. This helps to bridge connections in a patient's mind that they may not have thought of by themselves. It can also buy a little time for the practitioner in order to come up with the next question. At times, it is difficult to think of the next question. By giving feedback, it puts things into clearer perspective and the next question presents itself.

i) *Word for Word Feedback.*

Just as it says it is. A person says, "I don't like going to the zoo" and you say, "*You don't like going to the zoo.*"

ii) *The Essential Meaning Feedback.*

Translating or synthesizing all the words down to the essence of what they're saying without changing any of the meaning.

For example, a person says, "I don't like it that I have to pick up my children's toys and their clothes, clean up after them, cook for my husband and the kids, prepare the lunches, clean the house, take out the garbage and not have any time for myself." And you say, "*You don't like not having time for yourself and having to do all these chores at home.*" (If they say, yes, right, it can set up the next question that could naturally be, "*How does it make you feel to have to do all these chores and not have time for yourself?*")

iii) *The Essential Meaning +: the Essential Meaning Feedback put into even clearer context.*

This feedback involves some deeper insight than the person

even mentioned. It helps to bring them even a little deeper than what they stated. It helps to inject an element of clarity. This type of feedback remains on par with their own awareness, it is just a little deeper, clearer, and more advanced. Sometimes, it involves tying things together that they may have said separately and didn't recognize a connection. When done well, this can be effective at bringing things together for a patient and is another example of when using a little bit of direction can be helpful.

For example, a person says, "I am struggling a lot in my classes. I feel really stupid." And then they also say, "I am having a hard time with my boyfriend. He really frustrates me a lot because he doesn't listen to what I have to say. He thinks he's so smart. He makes me feel like I am not very smart." And at some other point, they mention, "My father always speaks to me like I am so stupid." So this sort of feedback could look like, *"You are struggling with your classes, and your boyfriend. You also said you feel your father speaks to you like you are stupid and that is also what you mentioned about how your classes and your boyfriend make you feel. So you are feeling the same way in your classes, around your boyfriend, and around your father. They all make you feel stupid."*

When I give a lot of feedback, I like to ask, *"Does that sound about right?"* Or, *"Does that resonate with you?"* because it is still feedback coming from me and I want to make sure I have that connection and recognition from the patient, who acknowledges the statement as true. Then it's back in their court and it's also like getting a green light to proceed. The next question here, for instance, (*a Reflecting Elsewhere question*) could be, *"Where did feeling stupid first start for you?"* Or it could focus more specifically on, *"What is it about your class and/or boyfriend and/or father that makes you feel stupid?"*

iv) *Incorrect/Inaccurate Feedback.*

This is a form of feedback that I discovered by actually making mistakes in feedback with my patients. A few times, I would give some feedback and it was inaccurate. Either I wasn't listening very well at the moment, or I had simply misunderstood what the patient had said to me and I gave them incorrect feedback. The result, in most cases, was remarkable. The patient pushed back with a much clearer and stronger expressing of what they were really expressing. So, for example, my incorrect feedback was like, "*So your boss doesn't listen to your ideas.*" And the response was "No! My boss makes me feel like a good-for-nothing!" Sometimes, misunderstanding someone can actually make them feel misunderstood and this causes them to dig deeper emotionally, on the spot, to answer more accurately and in a fashion that expresses what they are really trying to say. It's like a shortcut to the truth and it is normally quite spontaneous and real.

I don't suggest actually doing this purposefully because it does make it seem like you're not listening or paying attention. One shouldn't do this too often in any one dialogue. However, recognizing that incorrect feedback can still yield wonderful results, it takes a lot of pressure off your feedback and trying to get everything right and exactly what the patient said. So if you slip up from time to time or you didn't understand properly, don't worry about it. The result can still be quite positive.

Vis Dialogue Summary Until Now: So for now, in our understanding of the Holistic Counseling Dialogue, we have: **Ask non-directive questions, remember to go into and through the negative, go with the flow by asking the next question that naturally presents itself from the last thing the person said, keep to the context of the flow, reserve directive questions for key points, and occasionally give feedback.**

Part IIIB

More Complete List of Holistic Counseling Questions and their Purpose

Here is a more complete list of Holistic Counseling questions that can be asked. Keep in mind, there is no such thing as a complete list, since there are a multitude of questions that can be asked for any given case, and at specific times, we will find ourselves asking questions we've never asked before. But this is a thorough list of at least most of the questions one can ask. I have made the attempt to organize the questions in at least some order to help the left (logical side, which can be on the right for some) brain absorb the information, but really, a Holistic Vis Dialogue is not to be viewed as an organized trail from point A to point Z. I feel that the successes I have had with Holistic Counseling have been because I was able to ask any question at the appropriate time in a fashion which is very present with what the patient is currently saying, not based on any predictable formula. It's an improvisational dance. Any rigidity or need for predictability in practice will only interfere with the natural, live responses that arise from what the patient last said.

In Chapter 28 of this list, we'll examine the most simple, non-directive, open-ended questions, and also some more advanced questions and where they might be applied. In Chapter 29 of this list of questions, we'll look at more specialized questions and techniques and the surrounding situations that may call for them. In Chapter 30, we will explore the process of Holistic Counseling questions to get to the root cause through physical symptoms and disease that is in the body. In Chapter 31, we will examine the *Closing questions* as well as the surrounding situations that can arise when one encourages a patient to change their old belief patterns. In Chapter 32, we will examine ways of dealing with cases that are stuck or not advancing.

Most of these questions from any of the chapters can be applied at any point during the Vis Dialogue. The Holistic Counseling practitioner is called to be creative, flexible, intuitive, and ever-ready to improvise a question for the moment that they are facing with a patient. In the beginning, however, and if one feels unequipped to improvise and intuit the next best question, then one could go quite far memorizing this more complete list of questions, and getting a feel for the appropriate times where their application is indicated.

I will comment about the questions and answers in their respective context, to bring as much information forward regarding the questions, so that this list is not static and fixed, but breathes and communicates more than just a delineated set of words are able.

Chapter 28

Concise/Specific Questions

"How does that feel?"

This is a question often used in practice. One could do a lot for a patient simply by asking this question, over and over again. Of course that would get dull and repetitive, but still, by asking, *"And how does that feel?"* one can get quite deep with a patient.

For example, a person says, "I hate it when I am left out of things."

"How does it feel when you're left out of things?"

"I feel disrespected."

"How does disrespected feel to you?"

(this is definitely going into and through the negative.)

Or,

Slightly different question: "What does feeling disrespected feel like?"

"It feels devastating."

"What does feeling devastated feel like?"

"I don't know. It feels devastated."

When you hear a patient answer the same thing to a question as they did to the previous question, it's time to choose a different type question or a different way of asking it. I find it is common to ask the same type of question twice in a row, and maybe three times, but not more. As we will see, two or three flows nicely, and is often naturally well received, but as in chess, you shouldn't be able to make the same move back and forth more than three times.

Another question could be: *"What about feeling disrespected makes you feel devastated?"*

This is a question I would prefer to use in this instance, since I have already asked, "how does it feel" twice, and this helps to bring them to a more concise response. What is it about feeling disrespected, requires the patient to take a look at *what it is* about the feeling disrespected that makes them feel devastated. It will lead deeper because it is more concisely going into and through the negative. However, it's ok to ask a series of, "and how does *that* feel?"

Answer to the previous question: *"What about feeling disrespected makes you feel devastated?"*

"It's like no one respects who I am."

New Question: *"How does having no one respect who you are make you feel devastated?"*

So we have switched from just asking, "How does that feel?" to a slightly different way of asking it, which can subtly open up an avenue that was shut down with another similar question, or from asking the same type of question too many times in a row. Also, notice that I just asked the very thing they had said back to them to facilitate their deeper exploration of this issue.

"What does that mean?"

Remember, sometimes people do not respond well to, *"How does that feel to you?"* It could be that they judge any sort of emotion or feeling or are simply out of touch with the level of feeling. So this is an intellectual type of question which can be employed instead of, *"How does that feel?"*

A middle-aged woman with lots of anxiety around keeping things neat and tidy states:

"I am always rushing around to make things happen."

"What does it mean to make things happen?"

"It means to make sure that everything gets done."

"What does it mean to get everything done?"

"It means I am responsible for everything."

Aha! In this short example, a person has gone from stating that they rush around to try to get everything done, to declaring that they believe they are responsible for everything.

So the next question to employ here could be:

"What makes you think that?"

"What makes you think you are responsible for everything?"

"If I don't get things done, nobody else will do it."

"What makes you think that if you don't get things done, nobody else will do it?"

"At home. If I don't clean up, nobody else will clean up."

At this point, I will share another principle of Holistic Counseling that will help us follow the stream and not get caught up in a common difficulty we can encounter during the Vis Dialogue. In so doing, I will share some more advanced questions for this sort of situation.

The Blank-Stare, Open-Mouthed Wall – Keep on Going

This sort of answer (If I don't clean up, nobody else will clean up), I call a "blank stare, open-mouthed" wall, and that is not on the part of the patient, but on the part of the practitioner. It happens when a response from a patient seems so dead ended and obvious that it seems as if there's nothing to ask at this point that can get a person to go deeper. It occurs often in 'real' situations. For example, a situation may arise where we're dialoguing with a patient who got sick following the loss of a loved one. *"And when I lost my son, I knew life would never be the same."* Here, the practitioner can completely understand what the patient is saying and sympathizes so much so that there seems nothing else to be said or done. It can also feel like, "If I ask anything else right now, I will be so insensitive." It can make you sit there thinking, "Geez. I have nothing else to ask right now." The practitioner of Holistic Counseling must remember, that at all times, even though a real, tough situation exists, and what a person is experiencing is normal and natural, there are still other dimensions to be explored.

The patient is consulting you because of sickness and suffering. So yes, life is tough, and things happen that challenge us to the very core. But that doesn't mean that there have not been choices adopted that cannot be changed and released that are adding to our suffering. Therefore, in such a case, I will continue to press on with questions, to get to the bottom of the suffering. This requires a very strong and clear male energy balanced, of course, with compassionate and tender female energy. In plain terms, some real *chutzpah* is needed. If a practitioner has issues with "inconveniencing" others, if they feel hesitant to challenge others' pain, this part of the dialogue will be a stumbling block for them. Since this *blank-stare, open-mouthed wall* can be encountered often enough, it is necessary to do some deep soul-searching and to trust that, even when it seems so obvious what a patient is saying, there is always something else to be asked. Sometimes a person's response seems so "obvious" about the answer that one wouldn't think to ask anything about it. It's almost as if the patient is saying, "Don't you dare ask me anything else about this." Or, "This is point-finale, and there's nothing else to be said about this." This can be a little nerve wracking, but nevertheless, asking the patient about it can help them move past a story they've been telling themselves over and over that seems like the only truth, so obvious and matter of fact, as if there's nothing to be done about it. Don't stop there. Keep going. Keep investigating to find where the patient is holding onto the false belief that is making them sick. Once you've done this a few times, you'll have trust in the process and can go through it much less awkwardly when it arises.

Because of the great sensitivity we encounter at times where the real situation seems so obvious, I like to say the following to help the patient understand that I am not being, as it may seem, insensitive. *"I can only imagine what it must have been like to have lost your son. Your grief is natural and healthy. There may be something, however, that we can help you let go of that is not necessary for you to carry anymore and that has led to your health condition that you have come here to heal. So can we explore this further?"*

I have never encountered a patient that did not understand this once it was presented in such a fashion. They do want to heal. They do want to let go even if their grief has a powerful punch to it and they get angry when anything is suggested around letting it go. So when we encounter this sort of "wall," we press on. And remember, the wall can be related to any subject matter and any emotion.

So I may ask, *"What was the hardest part for you about losing your son?"*

"He was my light and my joy. Without him, there is no more love, no more light."

Again, we can totally understand someone deciding to feel this way following the loss of their child, but it nevertheless is a very conditional view of life and limits a person's reality, leading to illness.

"What makes you think that, without him, there is no more love, no more light?"

"I cannot imagine living without him."

Here, we could go a number of directions. One of the directions calls for a directive question.

"Do you want to keep on living?"

"Yes, but I miss him so much."

"So what would happen if you chose to keep on living and loving?"

(I added here, the notion of keeping on *loving* as well, because, just before, she had mentioned there is no more love without him. This is like feedback + where the practitioner ties something together that the patient didn't necessary say specifically themselves.)

"If I chose to keep on living and loving, it's like I would be saying that I don't love him anymore."

Aha! It is so interesting what can arise on the other side of a *blank-stare, open-mouthed wall*. This belief, evolving from her loss, and perhaps even having had some origins earlier in her life, is the false belief that she has become hooked into. It is limiting her life, her vitality, and has led to her suffering and health condition. So we would then continue to explore this belief at its present time in the stream of the dialogue.

And since this is such an important principle, we will now add it to our general summary of the Holistic Counseling principles.

Vis Dialogue Summary until now: Ask non-directive questions, go with the flow by asking the next open-ended question that naturally presents itself from the last thing the person said, keep to the context of the flow, reserve directive questions for key points, and occasionally give feedback, all the while remembering the important principle of going into and through the negative, and if a blank-stare, open-mouthed wall is encountered, keep on going.

So, back to where we left off just a little earlier in the previous case.

Question: *"What makes you think that if you don't get things done, nobody else will do it?"*

"At home. If I don't clean up, nobody else will clean up."

With the blank-stare, dead-ended responses, it's often a gutsy question that can be asked next.

Here's a new question. *"So what if?"*

So the next question could be:

"So what if nobody else cleans up?"

"Then they won't get done."

The answer could seem a little repetitive, or the person can have the attitude like "Duh!" but it doesn't matter. Keep pressing on with the questions, until you break through to a deeper level from which you would explore with more questions, or until a real dead end is arrived at, at which point you would go back and look for another question from a different angle.

"So what if you don't get things done?"

(Here is another example of how two questions of the same type were posed in a row. It's a natural flow emanating from the previous question.)

"If things don't get done, then the house will be in total disarray."

Here's a third time we can ask the same type of question:

"And what if the house is in total disarray?"

"Then it looks bad."

(Aha! So now, we've opened something up on a deeper level. Now, we are not just speaking about getting things done, but about how things will look bad if they are not done.)

Next Question: This most natural and 'following-the-stream question' –

"And if it looks bad? Then what?"

This is the same question as asking, *"And so what if it looks bad?"*

But since we've already asked that three times in a row with the same wording, I can mix up the words so that the patient doesn't start getting hypnotized by my repetitive questions.

"If the house looks bad, then I wouldn't want to have anybody over."

New Question: *"What about that makes you... do that, or feel that, or think that, or not want that?"*

"What about the house looking bad would make you not want to have anybody over?"

"I don't want anybody to think we're messy people."

"What makes you feel that way?" We could also ask:

"What makes you think that?" but it's not the most accurate or fluid question here, since the context doesn't match up. A more accurate question would be:

"What makes you not want others to think you're messy people?"

Or since they are mentioning something negative they don't want, you can always use the question:

"And what if they thought you were messy people?"

This way, we're going into the negative in the most simple and direct fashion.

"They'll think we're trashy people."

"What do you mean by 'trashy'?"

"You know. Like poor, trashy people. Like white trash."

"And so, What if they did think you were white trash?"

"I could not handle that."

(Aha! We are getting somewhere.)

A number of questions can be asked at this point:

"What makes you not be able to handle people thinking you were poor, like white trash?"

Or,

"What does it feel like to have people think you are poor, like white trash?"

Or,

Another question, that I can introduce now, is:

New Question: *"What does it bring up for you?"*

"What does it bring up for you, if people think you are poor, like white trash?"

All three of these questions would most likely lead to "Rome."

"It brings up the feeling of being like a good-for-nothing."

We could then ask, simply: *"Tell me about good-for-nothing."*

Another question we can do at this time is:

New Question: *"How does this make you feel or think that?"*

"How does people thinking you are poor, like white trash, make you feel like a good-for-nothing?"

(This is seeking to make a connection between the previous question and the latest question.)

"I don't know."

We will often hear people say, I don't know. It's ok. You can rephrase the question some other way to overcome a mental stumbling block.

"What is it like for you to have people think of you as a good-

for-nothing?"

"It's awful. It's so so very painful."

(Aha, so we're getting somewhere very deep now. Soon, we'll switch to a more specialized-type question to bring a broader perspective from just the current situation, to a larger, more global belief that is the thread that has run through the patient's life. That is what I call a *"Reflecting Elsewhere"* question. But for now, let's follow the stream.)

New Question: *"Tell me about..."* A simple way of getting a person to expand upon a thought or statement.

"Tell me about the pain you feel."

"It hurts so much. I try to avoid it."

We could ask here:

"What makes you try to avoid the pain?"

"I grew up and was told to grin and bear it."

New Question: *"What do you do with the pain/feeling..."*

This is a more advanced question asking a person how they deal with their woundedness, their pain and difficult emotions. The goal is to get them to realize that doing so is not in their best interest and is not healthy for them. Because of this, it is a sort of side track that is somewhat directional in nature, but we never know what tender spots will be exposed upon venturing down this path... will it lead to "Rome?"

"I stuff it down."

"What makes you stuff it down?"

"I grew up being told I shouldn't show my emotions. I should just grin and bear it."

(A simple investigative, following the stream question to bring more perspective at this point would be):

"Who told you that?" The answer can be revealing and helpful for the rest of the case.

"My father."

"Tell me about your father? What was he like?"

"He was an angry man. He drank too much and was very

lazy. The house where I grew up was always a mess. He didn't take care of anything and he made me feel like it was all my fault, because I was a girl. My brothers just got away with making a mess and they didn't have to do anything around the house. When I would get upset and cry, he would shout at me and tell me to stop and to grin and bear it."

Bingo! Here we arrive at a thread that reveals what makes this patient feel she is the only one responsible for keeping the house clean. We also came to understand that she stuffs down her emotions because her father would shout at her and tell her to grin and bear it. We also came to recognize that the house where she grew up was always a mess. This also points to her desire to not have it be a mess, and we can understand where the idea of being poor/trashy came from. Notice how the Vis works in this case. Because we had been following the stream, by opening up the subject of her father, she naturally continued to follow the stream and made connections about her previous statements and how they relate to her problem. Although she has not openly recognized the direct connection between the two, it is possible, at this point, our "spider sense" is tingling with the idea that she feels like a good-for-nothing because her father used to yell at her for not taking care of the house. Did he call her a "good-for-nothing" if she didn't keep the house clean? It's possible, but we should not assume. We can ask a question or we can also bring some feedback at this point to help establish that connection.

Once a connection has been established, that is an excellent time to bring feedback to the person to help them make the connection between the beginning of the dialogue, the places that were visited along the stream, and the deeper, more underlying feelings and beliefs.

Here we can ask:

"What were some of the specific names that your father called you?"

"He would call me useless, a good-for-nothing."

If the patient doesn't go "aha!" right now, you can do a little feedback, or do it all the same even if they did get an "aha!" moment. I often say, *"Say that again."* when a patient has just said something that ties things together without them realizing it. Or I will state, *"Let me say that back to you. "He would call me useless, a good-for-nothing." What does that sound like?"* That always does the trick when the patient's own "aha" mechanism needs a little oiling.

Here I give feedback:

"So you grew up in a house where your father was lazy and didn't do anything to take care of things. He also didn't expect anything from your brothers, just you." Here I will add a directive question to help make a connection:

New Question: *"Can we say...?"*

"Can we say that your feeling of being a good-for-nothing if something doesn't get done around your house nowadays comes from this situation with your father and your brothers, growing up?"

"Yes. Very much so."

There is one piece of the puzzle missing. The issue around not wanting to appear poor like white-trash.

"How does the feeling of being poor, like white trash fit into all of this?"

"I felt so embarrassed by my house. If I didn't take care of the mess, then I was worried that others would think we were white trash."

Aha! That ties just about everything together along the thread. More questions can be explored at this point to investigate what it would mean to her if people did think they were white trash. But for now, this is excellent progress. Later, in Chapter 31, we will look at what to do to help her with the underlying cause.

Let's go back a few steps to here:

"What is it like for you to have people think of you as a good-

for-nothing?"

"It's awful. It's so, so very painful."

The Vis Dialogue is very much like a *"Choose your Own Adventure"* story. Instead of pursuing the side-track about her trying to avoid her feelings, we could have pursued another road, which would most likely also lead to "Rome." The answers emanate from the patient, of course, but there is flexibility of direction, so long as we maintain the three most important principles of open-ended, non-directive questions, following the stream, and going into and through the negative.

Reflecting Elsewhere Questions

When we get down to a deep feeling, something very painful and troubling that is as a result of a present situation we're investigating, we want to get people to reflect upon another time or situation where they may have experienced the same thing before. It should be noted that not every patient will be expressing or experiencing deep pain. Some may be disconnected from it, or have been suppressing it for so long it is beyond their conscious awareness. Nevertheless, the practitioner will arrive at a deep, core belief which seems to be very foundational to the other issues at hand as well as the suffering in general. And so it is at this point where we can also ask one of several *"Reflecting Elsewhere"* questions. These questions are a little more advanced in that they lift the person out of the limited perspective of only one situation (i.e. not cleaning up in the present time), and makes them recognize the fact that they have struggled with this underlying belief or issue beyond the present situation.

So for instance, look back at this last dialogue where we got to this point:

"It brings up the feeling of being like a good-for-nothing."

Reflecting-Elsewhere questions:

"Where does this come from?"

"Where do you think you got that idea?"

"Have you ever experienced that before?"

"Is there anywhere else in your life that makes you or made you feel that same way?"

"What is your earliest memory of a situation that made you feel that way?"

So, if we ask her any one of the above questions, it will make her reflect upon the time when this started, or where it came from. This helps bring a larger perspective outside of the present situation and is a step or two deeper. It is also helping to illustrate a person's choice to have adopted a belief system rather than it just being a given. It points to a source of the belief system. If a person is stuck in suffering as a result of a deepseated, core belief, there is not much apparent choice in the matter. However, when you ask them, *"Where does this come from?"* and the answer is, "My father called me a good-fornothing," then we've set up an awareness that the very core idea itself came from somebody or somewhere else, beside the patient; i.e. they didn't create it. It was not supplied to them as the core DNA fabric of their I AM statement. It's like the dawning of awareness that I am not a toxic person. The water from the well I drank from is toxic.

"Where do you think you got the idea that you're good-fornothing?"

(after some reflection – we may need to give the patient some time to reflect):

"My father used to call me that."

"When would he call you that?"

"When I wouldn't be right on top of taking care of the house."

Here is an interesting point about trusting the patient and that The Healing Power of Nature lives inside of them. I've been surprised at how insightful patients' awareness can be into their own lives. I would say most patients make the connection following the *"Reflecting Elsewhere"* questions. Everyone has the ability to reflect and discover the connection between the present issue and another point in time that was the source of the problem.

Sometimes, patients cannot seem to make the connection. The wound may just be too buried or else they are getting in their own way. Often patients that are not able to take a stab at things like this are standing in their own way. The very belief system that is being explored is the very source of the problem that gets in their way. So, for instance, a patient can have a core belief that they are stupid. So, when you ask someone to make a connection, they will say, "I don't know" not because they don't know the answer, but because they have come to believe they don't know because they believe they're stupid. That is what stands in their way of just seeing the answer.

If they say, "I don't know," try to change up the questions a little, ask a different, yet related question. Here's another way we can go about this:

"Is there anywhere else in your life that made you feel like a good-for-nothing?"

"Ah. Yes. I do remember now. When I was younger."

"What was the situation like when you were younger that made you feel like a good-for-nothing?"

"My father would call me that when I wouldn't have the house looking perfectly clean."

So we just helped her to connect her present complaint – anxiety when she feels things aren't neat and tidy enough, to the source of where the beliefs and original wounds came from. This, alone, is very helpful and healing. Feedback at this point, can be given.

"So, you began by sharing with me that you feel a lot of anxiety when the house is not clean and tidy. When we explored a little deeper together, you said, that it makes you feel like a good-for-nothing. Then, you just said that, as a child, when you wouldn't keep the house clean and tidy, your father would call

you a good-for-nothing. Can you see the connection between how you're feeling nowadays and what your father made you feel when you were growing up?"

"Yes."

At this particular juncture in the dialogue, now that we have unveiled a very deep core belief, we should be ready to move into the *Closing questions*. We'll take this case example up later in Chapter 31 – *Closing Questions*, to examine the next steps to take to help someone change their mindset on what they believe to be true.

These next two new questions are also important questions for Chapter 30 – *Technique of going through the Physical Symptoms to get to the Root Cause*.

New Question: *"How long have you felt or believed that? When did it start?"*

In every case, this is a very standard and necessary question to ask, to establish when something began. Often, it is the very first question to ask when someone presents a physical symptom or an illness.

"When did you begin getting migraine headaches?"

This question presents the opportunity to explore what surrounding circumstances were present when the patient began experiencing symptoms of their condition or illness.

"About five years ago."

New Question: *"What was happening in your life at that time?"*

"Nothing special."

Patients will sometimes answer that nothing special was happening. That doesn't mean nothing happened that led to their illness. Usually, if not, most of the time, something did happen. They are just not yet consciously aware of it. This also occurs frequently in practice, and it is amusing to see when they make the connection and become aware of what had actually occurred that led to their illness.

At this point, I will ask a range of questions to toggle their memory.

"Did you have any troubles with a relationship? End a relationship? Start a new relationship? Did you have any acute illnesses, like the flu, pneumonia, fever, stomach flu, food poisoning? Did you injure yourself? Did you go traveling anywhere? Did you experience any traumatic events? Did you start a new job or go to a new school?"

More often than not, they will remember something that did occur at the time.

At this point, I will jump into a case that occurred during my clinical year at CCNM in 1999. The patient was a 25-year-old woman, with the chief concern of migraines. They had begun around 1.5 years earlier. It just so happened that her response to the question, *"What was happening in your life at the time?"* was, "Nothing special. I cannot remember anything happening in my life at that time."

I went through the whole slew of questions and no definite cause could be identified.

I then began asking her more questions about the headaches. They would begin every day around 1-2pm. I asked her what she did during the day. She responded that she worked.

"How do you feel at work?"

"Very stressed out."

"What stresses you out?"

"Upper management puts pressure on me to get the designers to finish their work. I am in middle management and my job is to get the designers to deliver their work to upper management. When they are behind schedule, I feel a lot of pressure from upper management."

"When did you begin your job?"

"Around 1.5 years ago." (Aha! Funny that I had asked her if she had begun a new job at that time and initially, she said no. But in this way, it became clear. People, sometimes honestly and sincerely cannot recall.)

"Isn't that when you said your migraines began?"

"Oh yeah."

So, being a 4th year clinician, I gave her a piece of advice. I don't normally do this anymore, now that I have developed a deeper understanding of the power of healing that comes from patients arriving at their own conclusions. I also had run out of time and could not pursue any further questions or homeopathic intake. I had just seen the movie *Seven Years in Tibet* starring Brad Pitt, and in the movie, there is a piece of Buddhist advice given by the Dalai Lama, and it went like this: "We have a saying in Tibet: If a problem can be solved there is no use worrying about it. If it can't be solved, worrying will do no good."[16]

She was extremely worried about the situation. Worry is a pain in the head, is it not? So, it really seemed clear to me that her migraines were being caused by this stress, even without knowing anything further. So, I quoted that saying in the movie to her, which was my piece of advice. I then asked her to come back the following week for a homeopathic intake. She missed the next week's appointment and showed up the following week, where she reported that she had not had one migraine since she took the piece of advice. It was a well-targeted idea that had actually addressed the cause of her migraines. She had been having a migraine every day of the work week for the previous one and half years and stopped when she decided to stop worrying about a problem she could not solve. It does demonstrate that sometimes, some well-targeted advice can lead to healing, provided the horse decides to drink at the waters of advice.

Here is another example of a case where we can apply this question.

It was of a 32-year-old woman with extreme anxiety and panic attacks.

"What would you like to address?"

"I would like to address the extreme anxiety that I feel."

"When did the anxiety begin?"

"Around four years ago."

"What was happening in your life at that time?"

"I had just gotten married and moved to my husband's home town."

So this a clear and big change in her life. Marriage and moving. From here we can investigate a little about how she felt about the change.

"What was it like for you to have just gotten married and to move to your husband's home town?"

"It was overwhelming."

"What part about it was most overwhelming for you?"

"Leaving my home town."

"What about leaving your hometown was overwhelming for you?"

"Leaving all my friends."

"What was it like for you to leave all your friends?"

"Very scary."

"What was scary about leaving your friends?"

"Moving to a new town where I didn't know anyone, except for my husband."

At this particular juncture, I could have asked a number of questions to help her make a connection between new town, and loss of friends. But really, the issue seemed to dwell with her loss of friends.

"How do you feel when you are in a town where you don't know anyone?"

"Very lost and alone."

(This could be a bit of an, "Oh yeah, I'd feel that way too" sort of situation. It's like a *blank-stare, open-mouthed* situation. And what do we do? Keep going!)

Now is a good time to ask the, *"What does it bring up for you?"* question.

"What does it bring up for you when you feel lost and alone?"

"A lot of anxiety." Aha! So we're onto something here, since this is her chief complaint, and we've found the scent that will lead to the source of her problem.

Now, we'll ask her a question to help her make a connection between her chief complaint and the situation. We can see, by this dialogue, a going into and through the negative, and also, very clearly, following the stream, from the last question she asked, to the next.

"How does feeling lost and alone make you feel anxious?"

(I'd like to inform the reader that some cases do unfold in a clear, step-by-step fashion, where each subsequent question allows the thread to unfold and to go a little deeper. However, it is not always the case, and in this case, it wasn't either. There was a lot of in between questions that didn't lead anywhere. However, these questions serve to "work at the knot" by pulling in different directions. Eventually, a question will open up a channel that leads deeper, toward the core. I have boiled down the questions that actually led somewhere. And I am illustrating the types of questions I used, and the situations where to apply the questions.)

"It's like, my friends aren't there to support me, so I feel anxious."

New Question: *"What does that give you?"*

(This sort of question helps to set up an awareness of what a person feels they need from the outside to compensate for a lack or deficiency of something on the inside.)

"What does the support of your friends give you?"

"They would give me feedback and a way of knowing if what I am doing is right or wrong."

(Aha! Wow. Now this is getting interesting. She began with describing her problem of anxiety. Then we asked when it began. When she got married and when she moved. I felt a twinge of an assumption when she told me that the anxiety had to do with being married. This was only my projection because as it turned out, it really didn't have anything to do with being married. It had everything to do with her relationship with herself, and how she felt without a close group of friends around her.

From this point on, I continued to question to get deeper to help her recognize what is really happening for her. This point was really just the tip of the iceberg, and the rest of the case unfolded in a very fascinating way.)

New Question: *"What if you did 'experience the thing you are afraid of,' what do you think would happen?"*

Remember, we're always looking for a way to go into and through the negative. One way to do that is by asking someone about how they'd feel if their fear, that they've just stated, did happen.

"What is frightening about that situation for you?"

Answer: "I could fail."

New Question: *"And what if you failed? What do you think would happen?"*

Any number of answers can come up. It all depends on the person and where they are with failure. Sometimes they realize, "Nothing. I guess nothing would happen." This is like getting to the basement floor and seeing there's nothing holding it up that has any substance. I discuss this further in Chapter 31 – *Closing questions.* Or they may say something like this:

"Oh failure is out of the question." (Many patients have a fear of failure. It is quite common. The big question is what is under-lying the fear of failure? It is like the fear of death. No one is really afraid of death, per se. It is what death represents to them that is most frightening for them. Loss of control. People forgetting about them. Who will take care of those dependent on me? (loss of role of caretaker.) Disappearing into a void of nothingness. Going to hell, etc.)

Here's a new case where fear of failure was a theme.

"What makes you think that failure is out of the question?"

"I've always believed that."

"Where does that idea come from?"

"From my dad. He always said, 'You never give up. Only losers give up.'"

"So how is that connected with failure for you?"

"Losers are failures."

Our new question reapplied now: *"And what if you were a loser?"*

Sometimes questions like this one can be quite edgy and touchy. If I sense that the patient is getting hung up on an edgy, touchy question, I will do a short and quick explanation to get past this stumbling block: *"Don't worry. I am not suggesting you are a loser and that you should accept that. I am just exploring with you what is behind the fear of being a loser. Is that ok?"* Remember the permission. A little bit of permission can go a long way. Most of the time patients understand the gist of these edgy, touchy questions and don't get caught up in them. It is when you sense they are struggling with the question itself, that you can give a little explanation as to what is making you ask it.

"If I was a loser, then nobody would like me."

"What makes you think that?" (Or we could also take the approach: *"And if nobody liked you, how would that be for you?"*)

Answer to, "What makes you think that?"

"Well, my dad and my uncles would laugh at underprivileged people, or people they thought were failures. They would call them losers."

"How did that make you feel?"

"I would feel so embarrassed for those people and I felt it was so condescending."

"Did anything like that ever happen to you?"

"Yes. When I played football. Once I didn't catch an important throw that could have resulted in us winning the game. After the game, my dad grabbed me by my arm in front of the whole team and my friends, and yanked me off the field."

"How did that make you feel?"

"I was so embarrassed. I felt so small and like the biggest failure. I felt like such a loser and like I had lost all my friends."

When a person expresses two or more feelings in one statement, I have found it most helpful, since we go into and through the negative, to ask which of the feelings has the most weight. We can also give a little feedback based on their question, within the next question, in case they forgot all the things they may have said.

New Question: *"So of all the things you just mentioned... you felt embarrassed, small and like the biggest failure. You also said you felt like a loser and like you had lost all your friends... which of those do you feel carries the most weight/impact?"*

"That I had lost all my friends."

So this is interesting. From asking him about his fear of failure, which was "out of the question," we have unearthed something hidden in his subconscious – a painful experience of failure that was embarrassing and where he felt like a loser. So the words that he had used earlier that had come up about his fear were "failure and loser." These are intertwined in a painful experience that wounded him. Also, the way his dad and uncles regarded underprivileged people is also somehow related. What is even more interesting is that what is most painful about that experience for him is that he felt he had lost all his friends. It wasn't the embarrassment that mattered the most. It wasn't the feeling of being a loser, or feeling small. It was the loss of his friends that had the most weight, the most impact. Those other feelings are other avenues that can be explored later if it seems important to do so. Or we can simply ask, at a later time: *"Tell me about feeling small and feeling embarrassed? Is that an issue for you?"*

"What was it like to feel like you'd lost all your friends?"

"It felt so terrible at first, but I later realized I hadn't lost all of my friends. Just some of my friends."

"Which friends did you end up losing?"

"Well, after that, Tim and Paulo weren't really nice to me anymore."

New directive question: *"Is that ok?"*

I like to ask the directive question *"Is that ok?"* to see if the person can see from a broader perspective and also to see how they regard the situation. If they are devastated, neutral or indifferent, or have a healthy response.

"I guess so. I ended up seeing a side of them I hadn't seen before. They weren't very nice guys."

Let's go back to our previous question to explore another form of questioning: *"What if you did 'experience the thing' you are afraid of."*

Someone says; "I feel I need to be perfect."

"And what if you were not perfect. What do you think would happen?"

Or as another example, someone says, "I need to be the rock of the family."

We can ask: *"And what if you were not the rock of the family. What is the worst thing that could happen?"*

I added, "What is the *worst thing* that could happen?" This is a good way to go into the negative and to get to the point of what is really troubling someone underlying their need to be in control, or to run from their fear.

Another way to word this question, for fluidity and flexibility, could be *"So... what would happen if you are not perfect? Or what would happen if you are not the rock?"*

Very simple ways to ask a person to elaborate more on something they've said.

New Questions:

"Tell me more."

"Go on."

"I don't understand what you mean by that?"

"Huh?" Yes. I do sometimes just say *"Huh?"* when I don't

understand a statement someone said. This can work just fine with some patients, and with others, I may use a more dignified wording.

"So?" sometimes a person states something and it is like they are making a statement without really spelling out what they are trying to say. I may say *"So?"* to get them to spell it out.

"And?" Sometimes people end a sentence and it feels like they have a thought which is ready to fall off the edge of a precipice, but they are not coughing it up, for whatever reason. Shyness. Fear to express the weakness. Fear to express their hatred. So I will say, *"And?"* to encourage them to state something further.

"When I go out in public, I don't like it when I am in a place that doesn't have visible exits."

"Go on." Or, *"Tell me more."*

"Well, it's like when I am in a crowd."

"And?"

"And there's no way out. I am trapped."

All of these simple questions can be used at different times. The reader can also gather from the simplicity of them and even the unsophisticated nature of them that it is not really about wording questions in a very fancy way, but to word the questions in the right way at the specified points in time during a dialogue that matters most.

New Question: *"What is the connection?"*

If you don't understand what a patient has said in response to a question that has led to something seemingly unrelated, ask, *"What is the connection between what we just discussed and what you just said?"* This can actually reveal some pretty profound workings of the mind, or perhaps it is better to state that as problems in the mind. Because when someone expresses themselves so that it is very difficult to understand, it means there is some sort of internal process in the person's mind that is not being shared. That is likely some form of belief or idea which is getting in the way of being communicated to the outside world.

Remember, we do not use the word Why in any question because it gums up the flow of the stream.

Vis Dialogue Summary Until Now: So for now, in our understanding of the Holistic Counseling Vis Dialogue, we have: **Ask non-directive questions, go with the flow by asking the next open-ended question that naturally presents itself from the last thing the person said, keep to the context of the flow, reserve directive questions for key points, and occasionally give feedback, all the while remembering the important principle of going into and through the negative and if a** *blank-stare, open-mouthed wall* **is encountered, keep on going. Ask** *"reflecting elsewhere"* **questions to help a person see their belief is not carved in stone.**

Summary of the Questions in Chapter 28.

"How does that feel?"

"What does feeling "X" e.g., disrespected, feel like?"

"How does having no one respect who you are make you feel devastated?" (Making a connection between two statements.)

"What does that mean?"

"What makes you think that?"

"So what if?"

"What about that makes you... do that, or feel that, or think that, or not want that?" e.g., *"What about the house looking bad would make you not want to have anybody over?"*

"What does it bring up for you?"

"How does this make you feel or think that?"

E.g.: *"How does people thinking you are poor, like white trash, make you feel like a good-for-nothing?"*

"What do you do with the pain/feeling..."

"What does that give you?"

E.g. *"What does the support of your friends give you?"*

"Reflecting Elsewhere" questions Part 1:

"Where does this come from?"

"Where do you think you got that idea?"

"Have you ever experienced that before?"

"Is there anywhere else in your life that makes you or made you feel that same way?"

"What is your earliest memory of a situation that made you feel that way?"

"How long have you felt or believed that? When did it start?"

"What was happening in your life at that time?"

"What if you did 'experience the thing you are afraid of,' what do you think would happen?" E.g: *"What if you failed? What do you think would happen?"*

"What is the worst thing that could happen?" E.g *"And what if you were not the rock of the family. What is the worst thing that could happen?"*

"So of all the things you just mentioned... which of those do you feel carries the most weight/impact for you?"

"Is that ok?"

"Tell me more."

"Tell me about..."

"Go on."

"I don't understand what you mean by that?"

"Huh?"

"So?"

"And?"

"What is the connection?"

Chapter 29

More Specialized, Advanced Questions and Techniques to Apply during the Vis Dialogue Process

Here are some more specialized and advanced questions that can be used to open up an obstinate case, or to get past some defenses that are difficult to budge. They can also be used simply because it is a very nice and appropriate time to pose these questions that will have the most naturally deepening response from the patient.

New Question: *"What's the opposite of that?"*

"What would the opposite feel like?"

Asking what the opposite of something is that the patient has expressed can yield a lot of information. Everything in Nature has an opposite. Yin and Yang. Day and Night. When we look at the Zodiac signs in the Heavens, they are also poised opposite each other. Mars and Venus, two opposites in Nature, exist on the opposite sides of the Zodiac. For example, Aries is opposite Libra. Aries is ruled by Mars and Libra is ruled by Venus. Mars and Venus are Yang and Yin to each other. Cancer is opposite Capricorn. Cancer is ruled by the Moon, Mother, and Capricorn by Saturn, the Father. *We can learn a lot about one sign by knowing its opposite*, in the other. For example, Taurus is about having things. Possessions. Stuff. Money. Whatever it may be. Taurus has it. They know they have it. It comes easily to them. Scorpio, on the opposite side of the Heavens, can get into desiring what others have. That is the opposite of the sense of Taurus.

So that gives us a good appreciation of the information we can get by looking into the opposite of something.

I often hear patients say how they would love to feel.

"I'd love to feel free, confident in myself, and able to take on the world."

"What is the opposite of that?" or we can also ask, *"What would the opposite of that feel like?"*

"Trapped, unsure of myself and very, very hesitant about everything."

Now we just check in to see if that is an accurate statement about how the patient feels, so we're not making any assumptions.

"Is that true for how you feel?"

"Very much so." That is a good confirmation. And it usually is the case when someone says the opposite of how they wish they were; that it is some form of negativity they experience.

We can also use "asking about the opposite" when someone is already describing how they feel in the negative.

"I feel gloomy and depressed, and I don't see any hope in anything."

"What is the opposite of that for you?"

"Happy and clear and that everything is ok. There's nothing to worry about. Everything is going to be fine."

"Do you ever feel that way in your life?"

"Yes. Sometimes I do."

"What is it that makes you switch between feeling happy and clear and that everything is ok to feeling gloomy and depressed and not seeing any hope?"

"It happens when I lose myself in a relationship."

Aha! This technique is designed to elicit an underlying understanding about what makes a person switch between their happy time and their not-so happy time. From here we could easily ask a number of questions. Some of the more plausible questions would be: *"How do you lose yourself in a relationship?" "Tell me about losing yourself in a relationship?" "What makes you lose yourself in a relationship?"*

And then the case will carry on from there.

(Note: something else here about the opposite. Another good

example, from a real case, perhaps, that illustrates when the best time to use this question is...)

Reflecting Elsewhere Question Part 2:

New Question: *"What is Common between these situations?"*

"Is there anywhere else in your life, or has there ever been another time that makes you feel this same way?" Put more simply: *"Where else in your life do you equally feel that way?"*

In the case shared earlier, a woman said she felt like her boyfriend made her feel stupid. This feeling of 'stupid' had a strong weight to it. It seemed quite painful and had a lot of charge and so most likely, it would lead to the core belief of the person. So I did some reflecting elsewhere questions with her.

"Is there anywhere else in your life where you are made to feel stupid?"

"Yes, with my boss and with my father."

A little feedback question: *"So you can feel stupid with your boyfriend, your boss, and your father?"*

"Yes."

Reflecting Elsewhere Question Part 2:

"What is common between these three situations?" Or we can ask: *"What is it about your father, your boyfriend, and your boss that makes you feel stupid?"* Part 2 of asking the patient to reflect elsewhere involves seeking the common thread or theme that runs through the time where they feel the same thing.

"I am not really sure, but I think it has to do with how I feel about them."

"How do you feel about them?"

"I really look up to them."

"What does that mean to you, that you really look up to them?"

"It means I think they are so smart, and I feel really small around them."

"What makes you feel that way?"

"I don't know. I've always done it."

"When is your earliest time that you did that?" (This is also a *Reflecting Elsewhere* question that looks for the earliest memory of a belief. This can show the source of the belief.)

"With my father." So now we see that the thread runs through her life with the boyfriend, the boss, and the father, but that it really began with the father.

"What made you do that with your father?"

"He was always so serious. If I did say something he didn't like or that he didn't agree with, I felt he just grumbled about it and he wouldn't say anything. He would stop talking to me. It made me feel bad."

"How did the feeling bad feel?"

"Like I was stupid or something."

"What made you think that?"

"I don't know. I just thought he must have not answered me back because what I said was stupid."

Here we can ask a number of things.

One question we can ask, *"Is it true that you're stupid?"* This is directive, a little bit of an edgy question, but works well nevertheless in the right moment. We can also ask it in a different way that softens the questions and still gets to the guts of the matter.

New Question (Reflecting on the past, which is related to *"Is it true?"*): *"Now that you're thinking about it, do you think that you were stupid those times when you said something he didn't like or agree with?"*

(This is also a directional question, and as we can see, this is another example in a case where we've gotten down to a sort of nitty gritty. We're working toward getting a person to see through the belief. We're looking to bring forth the awareness of the choice they are making. Here it takes trust in the person's ability to recognize the Truth about themselves. Most people can do this. Some are unable, only because of their particular woundedness. Either way, it doesn't hurt to endeavor to see what they'll say.)

"No. I actually don't think I was stupid."

The first thing that comes to mind is the *Closing question; "So do you want to keep believing that?"*

The answer is usually "No."

We can investigate this a little further.

"So what makes you choose to believe you are stupid now?"

"If I make myself small and stupid, then nothing I can say can make someone angry with me."

Aha! Now, this opens up something even deeper. By making oneself stupid, it prevents a situation that can make others angry. So it is not even really a belief about being stupid, per se, but a behavior she has done to prevent others from getting angry with her. It's more like she's convinced herself that she is stupid which has prevented her from seeing what she is truly concerned about – others being angry with her.

"And what if someone is angry with you?"

"Oh, I cannot handle that."

"What does it bring up for you if someone is angry with you?"

"It brings up the worst feeling, like I am falling apart."

"Tell me more."

"I feel I am falling apart, and I'll do anything to avoid that feeling."

"Like what?"

"Like making myself small and stupid, I suppose."

Here, we cycled back a little. We've essentially taken a step a little bit further up and out of the "Rabbit Hole," rather than deeper. It's ok because it ties in with what she said before, but this last question didn't actually help to go any deeper or further. So I'll then go back to where we were at the bottom line up until that point which was 'brings up the worst feeling like falling apart.' This sounds very negative. We haven't explored this by asking a question to go into and through the negative.

"Tell me what it is like to fall apart?"

"It's like my world is coming to an end."

"What is causing that?"

"When someone is angry with me."

"Yes, ok, but what is it about someone being angry with you that makes it feel like your world is coming to an end?"

Here the patient has a memory come up. This happens a lot when we're asking continual questions and getting deep into the subconscious. The original wound, or something that has contributed to it or is related to it, will surface.

"I remember once when my father got very angry with me. He stormed out of the house. I thought, that was it. He's never coming back."

"How did that feel to you?"

"Horrible. Horrible. The worst feeling in the world."

"How old were you?"

"Around 5 or 6 years old."

"Can you tell me more about how that feels? The worst feeling in the world?"

"Like I have done something that has the world come to an end."

"What did you do?"

"I made my father angry."

Aha! Now we have gotten the patient to declare something that has tied a few things together.

When someone is angry with her, it brings up the worst feeling. It reminds her of the time when she made her father angry and he stormed out of the house, leaving her feeling the worst feeling in the world. She had said earlier that this feeling is the worst feeling and she will do everything to avoid it, including making herself small and stupid to avoid making someone angry. That is her compensation and her way of running from fear. She makes herself small and stupid to *avoid* the feeling that she is so afraid of. So making herself small and stupid is the compensation. It may seem like it is what she wants, but it is just running from her fear. If I got stuck with her at this stage, I could share the *Two Paths and the Compensation* metaphor, but so far, there is no need. We're on a roll. We know a good part of the story, but there still may be a little bit more there. For instance, so what if he didn't come back? There may be something there. Nevertheless, it's time for some feedback.

"So making your father angry caused him to storm out of the house. You thought that he would never come back. This brought up the worst feeling for you, which you will do anything to avoid, including making yourself small and stupid so you don't make anyone angry with you. Is that about right?"

"Yes. Exactly right." (Tears shed at this point. The emotion is moving along with the awareness that is being unearthed.)

"Now what went through your mind when you thought your father would never come home because he was angry with you?"

"I thought he was leaving us for good. He was going to leave the family and it was all my fault."

"Because you made him mad." A kind of a feedback statement, question.

"Yes."

There are a number of avenues that could be pursued now. Here are some:

"What if he never came back?" We can ask this. It may lead to some underlying fears of being abandoned.

We can also ask, *"What if he left the family and it was all your fault?"*

We can ask the patient to reflect on what she thinks about the situation now. *"Now that you're looking at this situation again, from your present perspective, what do you think about it?"* This leaves it quite open for the patient to come up with whatever they feel about it spontaneously. If we want to be a little more directive, to bring a little more focus into a particular aspect of the situation, we can ask:

"Now that you're thinking about it again, do you think you'd really done something terribly wrong?" or, *"Now that you're thinking about it again, do you think it would really have been all your fault?"*

"No! I guess not. Sure, my father was mad at me. But he was always getting angry at everything. So, it wasn't me!"

This is a big shift for the patient, because this event seems to underlie a lot of her problem and her suffering. It, as a house of cards, is a lower level or the foundation of acting small and stupid to avoid the fear of causing someone to be angry. This is already a good time to bring in the *Closing questions*, to wrap up the situation. We've gotten to the bottom line. If this is not in fact the bottom line, ground zero, the foundation of the house of cards, when we ask the *Closing questions*, it will be revealed that there is a deeper underlying issue. But it does all seem to be resolved up until this point. The *Closing questions* are also intent on going back and asking if the patient wants to continue living that way, thinking or acting small or stupid. We would also ask her if she is going to continue thinking she has done something terribly wrong which is the end of the world. We'll take a closer look at the *Closing questions* later.

New Question: *"How is that working out for you?"*

This question is what I call a *"Transition question"* which we'll look at more in detail later. It's an excellent question that makes a patient reflect on whether or not the belief system or behavior pattern based on the ideas they hold is something that is good for them. In this case example, the patient says that making herself small will result in others not being angry with her. So it seems there is some motivation to her making herself small and stupid. This is her compensation and she is running from her fear of someone being angry with her. At that point in the dialogue, I could have asked her, *"How's that working out for you?"* Is she really invested in holding onto the idea of being stupid and small as a means of protecting herself from her fear?

Her answer would most likely be, as it often is; "It's not working out for me at all."

Many people laugh along with this question because they can see the absurdity of their belief. Most of the time, the patient is seeking help because they are sick and tired of the way their life has been, or they have gotten physically sick from an unhealthy belief and subsequent ways of being. So they are ready to let it go.

New Question: *"How did you respond to that? What was your response to that? How did you react to that sort of situation?"*

When we've gotten to a certain depth with a patient, and have come to understand a negative situation in their lives which has hurt them, it is important to find out what a person has done *as a result* of the negative situation. For example, in a case of a woman in her forties with multiple sclerosis, while I investigated how she felt about having the disease, she stated that she felt constricted, trapped, like there was no way out. The disease had progressed to the point where she was literally being confined by it to her house. She couldn't drive. Her sight was affected and she began having difficulty walking. I then asked her a *"Reflecting Elsewhere"* question – if there was anything in her life that had ever made her feel that way (trapped/constricted/no way out) and she said, "Yes, most definitely." She told me she had a very controlling mother, who would not allow her to do anything, nor decide anything for herself. She said:

"When in my senior year of High school, the colleges really begin courting you.

I was receiving all of this information from colleges and many invitations. I was already trying to formulate my own opinions – but my mother wouldn't allow that either.

So I was shut down right there. She wouldn't allow me to have my own opinion."

So here is where I would ask this sort of question:

"So what was your response to her not allowing you to have your opinion?" and/or another way of asking this: *"What would you do when she would shut you down and not allow you to formulate your own opinions?"*

That is the question which then allows a person to recognize what they began to do in their life which was not healthy for them. It also calls the choice out to the front. This particular woman's response was, "I did nothing. I just accepted it." I then asked:

"How did you then feel inside, as a result of just accepting your mother's control?"

This was a hard question for this woman to answer, because she had been so suppressed, and her mother's control over her had also included not allowing her to respond emotionally in any way, so she was largely out of touch with her emotional feelings and responses to her situation. But after persisting with many questions from different angles and worded differently to get at the feelings, she recognized that, because she didn't do anything to stand up for herself, or to fight against the control, she felt like she was trapped and that there was no way out. That was the thread for her which connected the past wound with her mother and what had crystallized inside of her and had led to her illness. And her illness had then manifested exactly that way, to the point where her life was beginning to reflect this "trapped" state of mind. She also had suicidal ideations, where she was feeling great despair. I asked her what the despair was like, and she responded, "Like there's no way out." She got to see all these links between how her very being was so suppressed and how, *by not fighting or doing anything against it*, she had come to feel like there was no way out and she was trapped.

Similar to the question, *"How did you respond to that?"* is the similar, but slightly different question: *"What do you do with that? What comes after that?"*

So you feel "x", for example, angry or sad or nervous, *"What do you do when you feel that? What is the next thing that you do when you're feeling angry/sad/nervous?"*

This is a good question that is handy to determine what people do as a result of feeling a certain way.

For example: *"When you feel angry, what do you do next?"* Or *"What comes after you get angry?"*

"Nothing. I shut it all down inside of myself."

This can lead to a number of exploratory questions.

"How is that working out for you?" (That is a *Transition question.*)

Or, *"Where do you think the anger goes?"* I've asked this exact question many times in cases, and I have yet to see one case not respond with A) it doesn't go anywhere. It stays stuck inside of me. And B) it is not good for them.

As another example, you can ask someone, *"So when you feel rejected, what do you do next?"*

"I want to isolate myself from everyone."

"What makes you do that?"

And exploration can continue from there.

Therefore, the question, *"What do you do next?"* helps expose a pattern in a person's life that is most likely repeated and predictable for them. The pattern is predictable because it originates from the wound and the person has a predictable way of handling the wound.

New Type of Question: "Can you see where you have misinterpreted something there? What would you have done differently?"

At the point in a case where a person recognizes the pattern, and where it came from, earlier in their life, and how they have chosen to respond to it, I will ask if they can see what their misinterpretation was during that situation. It helps them recognize the choice they have now to change. For instance, in the last case of the woman who was so afraid that by making her father mad, she had caused him to leave the family, which was the end of the world. By asking her, *"Now that you're thinking about it again, do you think you'd really done something terribly wrong?"* It is similar to this type of question, asking, *"Can you see how you may have misinterpreted the situation in the way you thought about it back then?"* That could have been an excellent approach in that instance as well. This is another example of a directive question.

Let's go back a step to the woman with MS whose mother wanted to control everything she did and said:

"How would you have done it differently now, if you could go back and change how you responded?"

This is also directive. One can see the usefulness at this point in the dialogue. There is a depth we have arrived at; now, the directiveness is designed to call into question an important decision to make in regards to the belief system. This woman with MS said: "I would trust myself more, believe in myself more, believe in all the other things people tell me all the times, how smart I am, talented... I wouldn't be as afraid of confronting somebody, or standing up for myself."

At that point, we would switch to a *Closing question*, which would be:

"What's stopping you from being that way now?"

New Question: *"What do you think/feel motivated that person to be the way they were with you?"*

I will also ask a person to consider/intuit what may have motivated the person that wounded them to have behaved in that fashion towards them. This serves a number of purposes. The first thing is that it really deflates the reality built up around that person as an authority of what is right and wrong. People often learn or adopt beliefs directly or indirectly from their parents. They often consider their parents as the ultimate, undeniable authorities on the Truth. When our patients take a look at what may have been the underlying motivation for their parents (or other friends, family members, teachers, etc.) to have been controlling and wounding, they gain a sense of wisdom about it and detachment. It is also a way of establishing compassion for a person's errors. Once compassion is established, acceptance and forgiveness can enter and this really helps a person move forward in their healing. For the patient, this technique/question also really isolates the choice inherent in believing in the reality that resulted from the control, from the wounding. If one can recognize that the parent or other loved one was coming from their own wounded place and their own "error", the patient's choice of whether or not to continue holding onto that reality as being truth becomes that much clearer and the letting go of it that much more permissible. And remember a most important fact about asking people questions. Sometimes, the answer is obvious, it is lying right there in the periphery of their subconscious, waiting to be revealed. But no one has ever asked the question, including the patient. So this is another form of the "gift of the right question." Had they asked themselves what may have motivated their mother/father to have been the way they were, they may have avoided quite a bit of additional pain and suffering. But they just never asked and they never were asked the question. Most people will have quite a profound insight into what motivated the parties that wounded them in their life.

One woman said her father was so controlling because he had been raised by his own father who was equally very tough and controlling with him. (That is often the case – a bloodline, sort of inheritance.) She also recognized that his most difficult life of toil, hard physical labor for many long hours every day, had made him bitter and too tough.

Another woman stated that her mother had kept her from feeling beautiful because she had learned from her own mother not to "let things go to children's heads." So this particular patient, with such a very hard time feeling good about herself, was wounded by her mother never saying anything nice and uplifting to her about her looks. Exploring this avenue with her was key in helping her recognize that her mother had made the same error that her grandmother had made raising her mother.

Another woman who struggled terribly with low self-esteem recognized that her father, who was the principle "wounding party" in her life, had a personality disorder, and her mother, complicit in her father's behavior, was trying to keep the peace and trying not to upset her father by not saying anything about his abusive behavior towards her.

Another woman who had issues with trusting herself, when asked what she felt motivated her father to behave the way he did with her, recognized that her father didn't handle emotions very well. When she was feeling emotional, he couldn't handle it. He would get very upset, act inappropriately and then blame his daughter, saying it was her fault that he was acting that way. This led to a pattern in her life where she didn't trust herself, the very thing she was consulting me for. She had been holding him in a position of authority in her mind, and recognizing that he was acting from a place where he was quite undeveloped emotionally and unable to handle her emotions, helped her have a different perspective on her original wound.

For each of these patients, the exploration of what motivated the wounding parties in their lives leads to a shift in awareness from "I am bad," "I did wrong," "It's my fault," to, "They were the ones to have made a mistake in how they behaved with me. I just misinterpreted that." Ultimately this helps lead to the freedom to decide no longer to live believing they were bad or that it was their fault.

The next few questions are techniques to ask questions from a different perspective.

Questions with an Observation:

"I noticed that you're (for e.g.) crossing your arms, touching your face, closing your eyes tightly, clenching your jaw, not

breathing, playing with your clothes, moving your feet back and forth? What's going on there for you?" or, *"What is making you do that?"* I use these questions when I am at a point that is a little stuck, just to help call more awareness to the patient in hopes of loosening the knot that is stuck. Remember, keeping the questions coming from different angles and perspectives is like pulling and working on a knot from different angles. It helps loosen it up.

When People Have Difficulty Describing their Emotional Pain

When people express that they are feeling emotional pain, sometimes it is difficult for them to describe it. They have trouble finding words for the pain. So we can ask different questions to bring about a focus, an awareness in hopes of eliciting a response regarding the pain.

"Where do you feel the pain?"

"Point on your body to where you feel the pain. What's it like in there?"

"Does the pain move around? Does it radiate anywhere else?"

"What colour is it? What texture is it?"

By getting a person to focus into their emotional pain and blockages, it helps that stuck, difficult energy to begin moving, which can bring about more expression and movement, to an ultimate release.

When People Express Things Vaguely: The Pot Metaphor

"How do you feel when you're put on the spot?"

"Bad."

"What does the bad feel like?"

"Terrible."

"What does the terrible feeling feel like?"

"Bad."

This is a funny scenario that can happen when a patient has yet to grasp what is the reason behind the questions. In such an instance, I will use a technique that I call *The Pot Metaphor*.

Here's how it works. I say:

"Imagine the "terrible" or the "bad" feeling is a pot, now throw it on the ground and let it all break open. What do you see inside of the pot? What is in there inside the bad and the terrible?"

Often this will work to get more information out of the person rather than just "bad" or "terrible." For example:

"It feels like turmoil. Like there's lots of turmoil inside of me."

Then we can ask: *"What does the turmoil feel like for you?"*

Remember, sometimes a person cannot answer a *"How does it feel?"* question because they are much more cerebral. So switch to a more neutral or intellectual question:

"Tell me about the turmoil." Or, *"What is the turmoil like?"*

If there's no response following the Pot Technique, or something related, we'll have to explore some possibilities in Chapter 32 on *"What to do when the case is not advancing or is stuck."*

New Question: *"What if you didn't believe that? What would your life be like if you didn't believe that?"*

These questions ask the patient to reflect on what their life would be like if they didn't hold fast to the core belief they take as their reality. So it can be used once the core belief has been brought out and the patient seems quite invested in it. They may have never thought of life without the belief or behavior before, and the idea is to invite them to consider what it would be like to live without their belief; this also beckons the idea of it being a choice, particularly to make the choice to change and heal appear more appealing.

For example: "I believe I always need to be the best."

"What if you didn't believe that? What would your life be like if you didn't believe that?"

"It would be much freer. I would feel much less stress and more relaxed. I'd also probably have more friends."

At a point like this in a given dialogue, we've gotten down to the bottom line (as far as we have discovered) and it is time to ask one of the *Closing questions.*

"So do you want to keep living this way?"

"No, but..."

When people are asked if they want to keep living the core belief, 99 times out of a 100, they will say no. I then estimate around 75% of the time, they will say "No, but..." and then express some form of doubt, fear, resistance, or hesitation about letting go of the belief. We will explore what to do with that in Chapter 31 on *Closing questions.*

Asking Two Questions at the Same Time

I've found myself often asking two questions at the same time. They are slightly different, one from the other, or they are the Yin and Yang of a question, helping to isolate the essence of a question by bringing in the query from more than one angle. The answer is then beckoned more from the essence of the questions, rather than needing to answer one or the other question. Or it can be that by providing two questions, one hits the spot better than the other. I do so rather spontaneously, as if I am reaching for an essential question which emerges as two. It is not like I am calculating two questions to ask. They emerge naturally, as I attempt to hit the nail on the head of the right question.

For example, we just saw two questions asked back to back:

"What if you didn't believe that? What would your life be like if you didn't believe that?"

One can sense how such a combination of questions calls the patient to reflect in a broader sense than just with one question. It's like a one-two punch. From the first question, the patient begins reflecting in that direction and then the second question brings them even further into reflection.

As another example:

"I am always hurrying everywhere. Rushing."

Two questions: *"What makes you hurry? What's pushing you to hurry?"*

Here the questions isolate two words, "makes and pushes" – sometimes, more than one word posed in the same question helps a patient find an answer because of having more possibilities.

As another example of this:

"I have this vague fear that seems to sit in the back of my mind all the time."

"What is the fear like?"

"I don't know. It's really too vague."

"What do you find yourself doing as a result of the fear? What do you feel you need to do when you're feeling the fear?"

The questions still work in harmony. They are not dividing the person's attention.

In a case I had of a man with myasthenia gravis and chronic fatigue, he said he knew at a certain point in his life that he could not turn back to the way things were, but also felt blocked from moving forward, like he was stuck in a sort of limbo.

So I asked:

"What stops you from moving forward? What is forward for you?"

It gave a fuller, broader question around forward, and left it up to the patient to respond. He ended up describing a situation that brings up the feeling of what not moving forward is about. It was an answer to the question.

In another case of a woman that had many problems that arose from her mother leaving the family when the patient was a very young girl:

"My mom told me, that even when I was little, 5-6 years old, when she would come to visit and then leave, I would be stone-faced, like 'whatever'. I wouldn't even shed a tear."

"What if you did cry? What do you feel that meant?"

"First thing that comes to mind, 'Don't let her know that she hurt you. Oh whatever, you're not important, I don't need you.'"

"What does that sound like?"

"Sounds like how I feel."

In another case, a man under a lot of pressure, suffering from depression, said:

"Now, I am more concerned, I just don't know what to do in terms of keeping my family safe."

"Safe from what? What is the threat?"

Don't ask two questions that make a patient respond to two different things at the same time.

For example: "I hate being interrupted. I wish people would let me talk. It's so disrespectful."

"What does it feel like being interrupted? Tell me about being disrespected?"

Those are two questions that work in different directions.

And don't do something like this:

"When did that idea of you being less than others begin? What would your life be like if you didn't feel that way?"

It's too divided in focus. Instead of doing that, just ask one question, follow the stream and then come back to ask the next question if need be, i.e. if the stream doesn't lead anywhere significant.

One thing that has been helpful is, at a certain point in the dialogue, I have two individual questions that won't work together if posed at the same time, but I do want to ask both, so I will say the following. *"Ok. I want to ask you two questions now. Answer whichever you'd like first, and then we'll come back to the other one. "What does it feel like being interrupted? What is it like for you to be disrespected?"*

This way, I don't forget what I want to ask and the patient can go with whichever question appeals to them the most.

Boiling down a Belief

Let's look at a case scenario to see how to help a patient "boil down" what they're saying into a belief.

This case example is of a man in his thirties describing anxiety at work. His main complaint is not being able to find what he wants to do in life. He hates his job but feels stuck, not knowing what else to do. He is struggling terribly with this and low self-esteem. He works very, very hard to ensure he hasn't made any mistakes. He will work twice as many hours, including after hours, to ensure his work is without any error.

We'll jump in the case here:

"I had a presentation with my boss and board members. I couldn't deliver what was expected...

In the end, it was horrible, my worst experience professionally.

I had to present – they thought I thought I was God and I should be the know-all and they attacked me...

At that time, I didn't know everything as well in the company.

"How did you feel about that?"

"I was devastated – I felt I was worthless, useless. I try to make sure it won't happen again, and it does anyway. Other times, I am put to the test. For example, next week I have to give a presentation to a room full of upper management.

I feel terrible. I can barely sleep properly. I feel weak, dizzy."

"What's the worst thing that can happen?"

"I don't look like I know what I am doing... or I am not competent, and my boss, who hired me to come there, will look bad, because it will look like she hired someone who was incompetent and I can give a bad name to the company."

"Which is the worst for you?"

"Good question. The first two – myself, looking incompetent and what my boss is going to think of me. What would be worse, is my boss, vs the upper management people."

"What is the worst thing that your boss could think of you?"

"That I am a fake and an idiot. I feel like a fraud."

"And if she did think you were a fraud? How do you feel about it?"

What is the worst thing?" (Here I actually asked *three* questions in a row.)

"I cannot stand sitting in a room and facing someone and the person thinks you're a fraud or an idiot. Them looking into me – thinking, I cannot rely on him or he is incompetent."

"Which is stronger or has more weight?"

"The incompetent one."

"So what if you are incompetent?"

"So... I don't know... You're worthless..."

"What makes you think you're worthless if you're incompetent?"

"I don't know."

(Now, at this point, I began boiling down the belief. This requires feedback and confirmation from the patient, to arrive at the most accurate version of the belief. Boiling down the belief starts with, *"Can we say?"* or something along those lines.)

"Can we say, one gains one's worth by being competent?"

"I guess. It doesn't have the ring to it, to say yes. But it's ok. It's close."

(He thinks about it for a moment and then says):

"Working hard is to be competent, and it is to maintain value and worth. Maintain value by being competent, not gain." (So the patient helped to correct the belief I had illustrated in a way that resonated more with him.)

"So can we say that if you feel you are not competent, you do not maintain your value and worth?"

"Yes. That is closer."

(Then he has an Aha! moment. He says the following in an excited, epiphany-like way.)

"I don't have value if I am not contributing to society in some helpful/beneficial way!"

This case was quite interesting. The patient was very insightful. As we went along, he discovered more and more beliefs about himself. I would boil down a belief, sometimes that was accurate, sometimes requiring some tweaking on his part. As the layers of beliefs were removed, we got deeper and deeper toward the source of his problem. The source of his problem, that is, "Rome," all stemmed from the fact that he was keeping his sexuality from his parents. Because of this, he felt like a fraud, and this was translating into other aspects of his life with "authority" figures, like his boss. Following our session, he summarized all the issues we had gotten through. He wrote the following and sent it to me:

I found my session with Dr. Moshe extremely helpful. It opened a part that I wanted to just avoid and forget about. (Being open about my sexuality to my parents), but seems to be one of the core causes to my other problems in life.)

To summarise the session, it seems we went down the following path:

1) I get dread, fear and nervousness at work and with dealing with persons of higher authority because I am afraid of failure and revealing that I am a "fraud."

2) I feel like a "fraud" because I am doing anything – even if I am not capable of doing it – just so I can meet a cause (environmental cause) and feel I have worth.

3) However, after realizing the worst thing that can happen to me is not losing my job or reputation – it's losing my parents.

4) I am also a "fraud" to them because I try my absolute best to hide my sexuality from them.

5) I fear that if they were to fully realize I am gay, it would kill them, and I cannot lose them because without them I would have no purpose in life.

6) Perhaps the reason why I don't know what I want to do in life is because I have always done what I thought was "right" but not what I really wanted. If my parents knew I was gay and

supported me knowing this, I am not sure where I would be right now.

This was very powerful for him to also see how the thread of feeling like a fraud that ran through his life stemmed from the feeling that he was hiding his sexuality from his parents, and pretending all the time; that made him feel like a fraud. He hid from both of his parents, but mostly, his father, who was the most authoritarian, "macho-type" man in his life. So, in the face of authority, he felt like a fraud, because he felt like a fraud with his father, who was the principle and original figure of authority in his life. This is another example of sympathetic resonance between two similar things, and shows how to follow a thread to find its source. This helps to unravel the issue. Later, during a subsequent follow-up, he realized that his father never helped him feel like he was ok just as he was. As a young boy, he identified strongly with his feminine energy, and his father and his mother, both, would discourage him from being effeminate. His father would say things like, "Oh, stop that! You look like a faggot." He began needing to hide from them to "survive" and he discovered that his desire to do something useful/beneficial in society was so that his father would accept him and think he was worth something. This is his compensation. This had led to his great confusion and unhappiness in his work life. He had been trying to win his father's approval by doing something that he thought his father would find helpful and useful for society. It was not what he wanted, but what his father wanted. All of this was mixed up with the fear of losing his parents. Because, he felt, that if they ever knew he was gay, it would kill them. A very interesting case.

Next case:

Here is another case of a woman in her thirties who had a very hard time expressing herself. She also had an issue of always trying to help people and to save them from their problems. She would do so by offering helpful advice. In this case, I help her to isolate what she is doing with this technique of boiling down a belief.

It began with the scenario of saying how she would go over and over thoughts and prepare for a coming discussion that could be confrontational, and then she would just not say anything during the conversation.

I asked: *"What would stop you from saying what you prepared months or days for?"*

"I start to imagine everything that could go wrong and then I start to just – If this goes wrong, this or this may happen. I always think of the negative instead of the positive. Then I get myself all worked up for what might happen. And then I say nothing."

"What stops you from saying something?"

"It's always in a bit of a confrontational situation. I have to go and disagree. That has been hanging over me for 3 weeks and I keep putting it off. What if I say the wrong thing? What if I am not strong enough to hold my stance? What if I cave in? This happens with my ex. And even forgetting – what if I forget all of my good reasons for this and for that? It drains me when I get into those situations. It's so draining. I do find, when I just do it – whatever I was putting off due to fear of confrontation, saying the wrong thing, it turns out fine. But with my ex – nothing ever does turn out fine. That has hung over me for years and years and years and it is a huge source of what drains me – disables me from being totally happy."

"Having stuff to say and not saying it?"

"Yeah."

"How does it feel to have stuff to say and not say it?"

"Frustrating."

"What is your earliest memory of having stuff to say and not saying it?"

"First thought was high school. I was also feeling that pressure to be responsible for everybody. Everyone's problems."

"What was common between then and now?"

"It is because what I have to say doesn't matter." (I could have asked now *"What makes you think that what you have to say doesn't matter? Where does that come from?)*

Instead, I asked:

"Where does the pressure to be responsible for everybody come from?"

"It's because when I am helping someone else, what I have to say matters, but when I have to say something for myself, it doesn't seem to matter to anybody. I don't feel that way with my friends, but it feels like it keeps coming up elsewhere in my life."

(Her answer was very profound and actually helped to link between the issues of being responsible for everyone, and also, what she has to say doesn't matter. I felt guided to ask about the pressure to be responsible for others because it felt like a stronger direction which would help go deeper. But had I asked about 'what I have to say doesn't matter' it would also have led to "Rome.")

(Here is where I help to boil down/isolate the belief. It is a kind of feedback.)

"So can we say that feeling responsible for everybody is a way of compensating for feeling like what you have to say doesn't matter?" (She just about said it in plain words as well. This is to help crystalize what has been said. It's not much of a jump at this point. It is a form of feedback +.)

She then says:

"Yes. I compensate by helping others so I feel what I have to say matters to compensate for feeling like what I have to say doesn't matter."

This was a big breakthrough that unified two keys issues. Being afraid to express herself, and also feeling a lot of pressure being responsible for everybody.

Next Case:

The next case is of a woman in her 30s with pretty severe psoriasis.

After asking many questions, we arrive at a point in the dialogue where she expresses that she never felt loved by her parents. This is what many of the issues in her life seem to be boiling down to. And I encounter the blank-stare, open-mouthed wall a few times with her, likely as a result of the severity of her pathology. Yet I continued to press on.

She said: "I think my parents think I am self-sufficient. 'She doesn't need it as much as the others do.' I took off and went around the world. They figured, 'She is ok. The other ones are more needy.' But it's not the case. I've said that to my mother – I need you too."

"What do you need from your mother?"

"I just need to know she cares about me. I need them to be on my side. To care for me, to nurture me."

"What if they don't ever care for you or nurture you?"

"It is what I have experienced for most of my life. It is always what I can do for them.

They don't call me up just to say, 'Hey, I love you, and we're interested in you.'

I always play the role of pleaser, rather than being nurtured."

"What does it give you to know that she cares about you?"
(She doesn't really answer this at first.)

"When I graduated, I had to fight to get my dad to come, because he didn't want to come!!

There's no… it's like having to fight for him to come. I am your child, why do I have to fight for your affection? My mom said, 'Yes yes yes, you did it!' She was so emotionally happy for me.

I was really struck by that. There was only one other time she did that. She was so proud of me. It gives me validation when I know they love me. Makes me feel good about who I am. Makes me feel good about who I am."

So here, I boil down the belief with her.

"So can we say: I feel good about who I am, and I let myself feel validated, when I know that my mother cares about me?"

Her response is:

"I feel I'd never have to go and shop if I felt I had all the support underneath of me. To feel validated. My worldview would change –world would not seem hostile. It would be friendly and amazing and supportive."

"What makes you need to get that from your mother and dad?"

"Because they are the pillars. They are my parents. It's the foundation of my life. My parents are the pillars. If I had them loving me and nurturing me the way I hoped for, it would be very different for me, versus I feel I have to pull teeth to get love. And having that unsecured foundation makes me feel I cannot be as free as I want. And there, I need to go get all that other stuff I do because I didn't get it from them. It's like there's a big hole in the foundation and I need to fill it with other stuff."

"How does it work to fill the hole?" (A *Transition question* which is like *"How's that working out for you?"*)

"It sucks, it doesn't work."

Then I boil down the belief again, with the additional information I have.

"Can we say this: Without the secure and clear love and nurturing and support from my parents, I do not have any foundation of support in my life and so life is a scary, uncertain thing?"

She says, "Yes, and I don't feel good about myself, because that same love acts as a validation for me. There are times when they will say, 'I am proud of you.' Oh, they said they loved me, they said they were proud of me."

"What does it give you?"

"It gives me confidence and makes me feel good about myself. It's because it is a validation. That I am worth loving and I am good person and I am doing a good job."

"If you never got it from them – what are other options?"

"I try to get it from other people. I know this way doesn't seem to help. Because then I put all the expectations on my parents on other people."

"Any other option?"

"Or I try to find it within myself."

"What happens when you do that?"

"That is where I keep coming up against the false belief. Where I am not worthy. I try to tell myself, I am worthy. So I found it difficult to change those beliefs, because they have been externally validated by the lack of love I've received."

"How has that validated you are not worthy of love?"

"Parents are your teachers. My teachers taught me that I wasn't worthy. It's going back to rewrite that – me saying, 'No, that is wrong. You are validated, just for the sake of existing.' I have a really hard time believing that."

(Here I boil down the belief again with her.)

"So can we say that you believe:

Your parents are the pillars, the foundation and the teachers. So what they establish with you becomes your reality."

"Yes. I fight that as an adult, but for most of my life, it has been the truth."

"Where does that idea come from?"

"It comes from my upbringing and it was all I had."

(Then she says something which I find interesting. It sticks out as not being a real continuity or making sense. This is something important that needs to become the focus. Because, like in homeopathy, just as we look for the strange, rare, and peculiar symptoms, this is a strange and peculiar thing to say, in a sense. So it needs to be explored.)

"I love them. They are my parents. Because they are the authority. They are the ones I would measure what is right and wrong for me."

(So what struck me as odd was *how* she said "I love them. They are my parents." It sounded almost as if she was saying, "Because I love them and they are my parents, I have to believe what they have established with me as reality.") So I ask:

"Where did you get the idea that what they say is so important?"

"I don't know. It has always been that way."

"Do you want to continue believing it?"

"No!! But I am afraid that that means I don't love my parents anymore."

(Aha! This confirms what I "heard" her say between the lines before. Here she states it again – that somehow to challenge what her parents said means that she doesn't love them anymore. It's a strange notion. She fills in the belief between the lines of that strange and peculiar thing she dropped in just earlier. It looks like we are getting to a core which is even deeper than we have ever gotten before.)

She continues:

"Because I do love them and want a relationship with them. But I know they will never love me the way I want to."

"What makes you think that not believing your parents are the authority and the pillars and your teachers means you won't have a relationship with them anymore?"

"I fear if I have to let go of those beliefs, then I have to let go of my parents. If I reject those ideas, I would be mad. If I reject those ideas, I would reject them. I'd be in opposition."

"To the ideas or to them?"

(And now she says something very profound.)

"Just to the ideas, because my parents love me."

(This is something profound that we see when we begin to "loosen" the hold a person has on their beliefs. They spontaneously begin asserting a different view which is more healthy and more true. Initially, and for a long time, she has felt that her parents don't love her. Then, when we get to this core belief, that challenging her parents' beliefs means not loving them, and not having a relationship with them, she says that her parents actually do love her. It is a sign of spontaneous healing.) Then she says:

"So it's just a big chip on my shoulder that I have to let go of because they do love me. But I understand they love me, not the way I want, but I can love myself enough that that is all that matters. I just don't know how. I don't know how to do it. Can I teach myself how to do this?

Yeah. I don't need to keep looking outside myself for everything. The idea was – If I take away their authority that means I don't love them. To love them is to give them authority. When it is not true. I can just love them for who they are. And love myself for who I am."

This represents an excellent awareness and something she had not stated earlier. It shows a real triumph in her healing, by moving past this most deep stumbling block (of a belief system) she was not able to move past. One of the most potent beliefs in all of this was, "If I remove the beliefs they taught me, it means I take away their authority and *that* means I don't love them." It was a great stumbling block for her because she believed that if she changed the foundation of reality that came from her parents, it meant that she didn't love them and she didn't want to stop loving them, nor stop from having a relationship with them. So this made her stuck into believing in whatever reality they had established with her, which, she had believed, was that they didn't love her. By seeing through this belief, it allowed her to stop giving her parents authority of whether or not she was lovable, and allowed her to switch into loving herself.

Isolating Conditional I AM Statements

This technique is similar to the previous one where we helped to boil down beliefs for the purpose of clarity. Working to isolate conditional I AM statements can be very helpful. Our I AM statements are statements of creation. They are ideas that emerge from our soul and guide the very fabric of our being. When our I AM statements are a reflection of our soul and our true nature and we are allowing ourselves to live by them, we are healthy, happy,

and free. When an element of conditionality enters the picture of our I AM statement, we become limited and restricted to creating ourselves in a way other than our true nature. This leads to disease and unhappiness.

Patients will not word their conditional I AM statements in such a clear and obvious way. That's why we use this technique to help them come face to face with what they're really saying about themselves.

Rene Descartes' famous statement "I think, therefore I am" is an example of an I AM statement. In fact, it is also conditional as the basis for an I AM statement. Because, what if I am not thinking? What if I am in a state of pure I AM consciousness? I still AM, am I not? Do I need to think, to be? No. I don't. So, "I think, therefore I am" is in fact, a conditional I AM statement.

When a patient is so very conditionally dependent on some form of control or need from the outside world to fulfill them or give them the apparent right to exist, we can use this statement with them.

For example, a man says, "Without a good job, I am nothing."

Question: *"So can we say "I have a good job, therefore I Am?""*

As another example, a woman says, "If I don't have children, I have no reason to be."

Question: *"So can we say, "I have children, therefore I Am?""*

And with another example, a man loses his position as a very prominent religious leader in his society. He says, "Without my position as a religious leader, I am nothing. Life is pointless now."

Question: *"So can we say "I am a religious leader, therefore I Am?""*

Or we could also ask: *"So can we say "I am a prominent person in society, therefore I Am?"*

In one case, a man in his sixties with myasthenia gravis was having a hard time walking around and spending quality time with his wife and children. This was such a horrible stress on him that he spent a good portion of every day worrying about it and it was eating him up. He said it was killing him.

"My wife is a very loving lady. I want to give back, but cannot. So I am buying stuff for my daughter, because I cannot give her anything else. So she has a smile on her face."

"What if you cannot give to your wife and daughter?"

"There's no point of living if you cannot do this. What's the point? Why we live? To make money, get drunk, get high? I am more spiritual than that. The only reason I am fighting for green, to pay my bills. I am not greedy. I don't want to build empires. Just fighting to pay my bills to take care of my family. If we cannot give love, I don't see the reason for that existence."

So then I stated the following:

"So can we say, "I provide for my family – therefore I am.""
"Yes."

In all of these examples, we're helping a patient realize they have stacked all of their eggs of their I AM statement, into one small, very conditional basket. This is very limiting. Isolating the conditional I Am statement helps to bring a perspective to their thinking that they may not have realized. It often calls to mind the sentiment "Yes, I have been thinking that, haven't I? It's very limiting, isn't it?" From there, we can move on to some *Closing questions*, like, *"Do you want to keep believing that your I Am statement about yourself is dependent on... having money, having children, being a religious leader, being a provider?"*

More on this in Chapter 31 on *Closing questions*.

Take a Guess Technique

This is a technique that I use all the time when a patient answers "I don't know" to two or more questions in a row. When I hear one "I don't know" to a question, I will try to ask a number of other questions to see if it gets past the person's "I don't know" defense. And it is just that – a defense or a barrier from the person being in touch with themselves. People have the answers. They are living children of Creation. The Truth lives inside of them, but they have become disconnected from the Truth. In the process, they have set up all sorts of mental traps, labyrinths and knee-jerk resistance patterns to avoid having to face the truth. The Truth always sets us free and is healing. However, as we've discussed in previous chapters regarding looking for the candy behind a person's illness, or *Compensation and the Two Paths*, people do become invested in not healing, and in not knowing what is going on for them.

A person is in an unhappy relationship but they are afraid to end it because they fear being alone, so they begin ignoring their thoughts and feeling about the relationship. In comes the Vis Dialogue:

"What makes you ignore your feelings in the relationship?"
"I don't know."
"Well, what do you feel right now thinking about it?"
"I have no idea."
"What stops you from expressing how you're feeling in the relationship?"
"I don't know."
Ok. So here is a good time to use the "take a guess" technique.
"Take a guess. What makes you ignore your feelings in the relationship?"
"I don't know."
If the patient says this again, then I'll say; *"It's ok. There's really no right or wrong answer. Just take a guess and we'll see what comes up."*
"I am afraid to see what I am really feeling."
"Does that answer feel right to you?"
"Yes." (Always check in. Then we can continue with the questioning from there.)
To the checking-in question, they may say "I am not sure."
At which case I would say, *"Well, let's ask a few more*

questions and see if it goes anywhere."

"What makes you afraid to see how you're really feeling?"

"Because I know what I am feeling and I don't want to face it."

"Does that feel right?" Or, *"Does that resonate with you?"*

"Yes. Definitely."

At this point, you can, but don't have to, confirm that the guess was in fact correct.

"So, was your guess accurate?"

"Yes."

Of course, from this point in the stream, we could ask one of two questions:

"What are you feeling that you don't want to face?"

Or:

"What makes you not want to face what you're feeling?"

"Because I know I don't really want to be in the relationship but I am afraid to leave."

From here, we can explore, through the Holistic Counseling Vis Dialogue, what is behind their fear to leave.

And this is the key to this technique – getting past a person's defense. A person's rational mind gets in the way and thinks or projects *not knowing* onto a situation. When we ask someone to guess, we are not asking them for the right answer. There is no pressure to come up with the right answer. It's just a guess, so how big a deal can it be? This lets the rational step out of the way which enables a person to answer from their instincts. Most of the time, the guesses do yield positive results. And once the rational defense and resistance has been bypassed then we ask for confirmation on the validity of the guess.

Chapter 30

Technique of Going through the Physical Symptoms to Get to the Root Cause

This is a very important chapter and deserves a lot of attention. I rarely get cases that do not have physical disease as the chief complaint. This technique helps to not only get to the root cause, but also helps to resolve the physical pathology. People often think counseling is for mental-emotional issues only and wouldn't think of going to a counselor for their physical disease. Never underestimate how far a person's perceptions can be from what the scope of practice is for a Naturopathic doctor. I've had people that I work with for myasthenia gravis say they didn't think of referring a friend to me because she had depression. I've also worked with patients that had mental-emotional disorders that I helped tremendously with Holistic Counseling say they didn't think of referring to me someone who had physical illness because they thought I only worked with counseling. It's important to be clear about this to people. It is also my hope that more and more people will come to recognize that their physical disease can be helped and even cured through the Holistic Counseling process. I've seen many cases of physical disease, including the allegedly "incurable" disease of myasthenia gravis, improve and even become cured with nothing else but the awareness and change of beliefs that came through the Holistic Counseling Vis Dialogue. The more we understand the mind-body connection, the more we trust The Healing Power of Nature and the laws of Nature cure, the more we can really see the diseases that are embedded in a person's body are the crystal-lized, physical form of the illness that began in their distorted perception of themselves and the world around them. And with that, and time, and patience (although some cases heal very fast once the belief is released), we can help most physical diseases that we encounter.

When I begin a case that has physical disease, or with physical symptoms as the chief concern, I will always begin by investigating the physical aspects of the disease. I do this because many people tend to be skeptical regarding the mind-body connection. They are coming to this new doctor's office for a disease and the doctor begins asking them about their mental-emotional symptoms. Like... huh? Even though I do have people read a PDF document that I have prepared for what to expect when working with me, there is something very special that occurs when we begin with the physical symptoms. People feel like they have been well-listened to. Their complaints and physical suffering has been well-documented. But another thing occurs that is much farther reaching than either of those previous points. And that is the witnessing of the mind-body connection by the patient. It is much more potent to begin with the physical condition and to have a patient express a metaphor for how it feels, or what it makes them do, or not do, and with specific words and phrases. Then, when they hear themselves use the same metaphor, words and phrases relating to some aspect of their lives at large, or their beliefs, there is a great "aha!" bright light moment, when they recognize the connection. And this is how it should be, because the body is a faithful puppy dog for the mind, and those beliefs and emotions that are not in harmony with a person's I AM, do get stored and crystallized into a person's body, including organs, muscles, bones, nervous system, and other tissues.

So to begin with the physical symptoms, it becomes clear soon enough that there is a lot more to this condition than the physical symptoms themselves. People use expressions and describe their physical symptoms in such a way that begs to be explored in the mental-emotional realms. For example, a patient says about the cramping pain in their legs; "I feel like something is holding me back." Or for someone with a thyroid condition states, "I feel like there are two hands around my neck choking me."

The way to start Holistic Counseling with a physical symptom, or disease, is rather simple. We ask everything that we can possibly think of asking about the condition. Such a thorough list of investigation is useful for homeopathy, as we will not want to come back later, after a big breakthrough near the end of the session, to begin collecting little bits of information regarding a condition that we have just "broken open" in mind-body awareness. The information can also come into play in unusual ways during the connection between the mind and body. Little nuances of the symptoms and triggers can make sense once we understand the underlying issues that reside within the person that led to the illness. For instance, everything is worse around the full moon definitely points to a lunar influence of the case, as well as a potential connection to the mother, as the moon rules the feminine and in particular, the mother. Another example of a special nuance could be that the pain is mostly on the *right* side, and we see later that it relates to how he feels about his father. The right side is related to the male energy and the left, to the female. And then there are the things that make the condition worse, which can be investigated to discover what is underlying the case. For example, in a particular cause, the complaint is worse at work. *"Well, what makes it worse at work?"* Surely, not "work" itself. That is too vague. *"So what really is making it worse at work? The cramped chair? Staring too long at a computer? The pressure? The boss?"* I consider we Holistic Counselors as "Detectives of Nature." That is what we are. The sleuths of the healing world. We ask questions to reveal clues to a deeper pathway that leads to the culprit behind the disease.

I suggest leaving the questions like, *"How does it feel? And how does it make you feel?"* for the last of the exploration surrounding the physical pathology, because it is mostly through these last questions that we will then begin connecting with the larger life "picture." If we begin to jump into the larger picture without some of the basic background information relating to the physical pathology, we may be missing some valuable information for later.

Here's a good list of questions to ask about a physical symptom or condition.

Questions to Investigate a Physical Condition or Symptom

E.g. Headaches – chronic

Begin with the Basic, Mundane Questions

"When did it first start?"

"What time does it come on? How long does it last?"

"What activities or situations bring it on?"

"Quality of the pain? Severity from 1 to 10."

"What makes it better? Worse?"

"What else accompanies the symptoms?"

More Advanced Exploratory Questions

"What was happening in your life when it began?"

"How does it feel?" (By asking how the pain or the symptom feels we can get to the underlying emotional/mental state that led to the symptom.)

"How does this affect your life?" (This is related to the next question.)

*"How does **make you feel?"* Or, *"How do you feel about it?"* (This relates to the section in Chapter 30 on *The way someone feels about their illness/what they think about it, what it makes them do, or not do, is a reflection of what got them sick in the first place.*)

After beginning to engage in these more exploratory questions, when something begins to sound like it could actually be referring to a situation in life, a feeling, a relationship, then ask: *"Where else in your life does this happen?"* Or, *"Is there anywhere else in your life that makes you feel this way?"*

(*Reflecting Elsewhere* questions to create that bridge between inner worlds and outer worlds.)

Important questions for going deeper:

"How does it feel?"

"How do you feel **about** *it?"*

"How does it **make** *you feel?"*

The important questions for going deeper are the bridge questions that will begin to open up a connection between the physical manifestations of their condition and the root cause. They are each subtly different, yet the latter of the two are more similar than the first question. Take a moment to reflect on the differences and similarities between these three questions.

Related to when it began: ***"What was going on during that time?"***

A major question we use in connecting the mind and body, and also, the beliefs to the origin of the disease is, after we have asked them when it started, to then ask, ***"Was there anything that happened out of the ordinary during your life right around or just before that time that you got sick?"***

And just as we used the *"Reflecting Elsewhere"* questions in Chapter 29, so too will we use those questions to bridge between the body and the mind. Once we get a person to express their condition where it sounds like they are describing a social situation, a relationship with another, how it might be at their job, etc., then we will pose one of the key body-mind connection questions: ***"Is there anywhere else in your life that makes you feel that way?"***

Case Example: 62 year old woman with chronic, painful kidney stones.

(Remember, I still have been condensing the cases to illustrate only the questions and the technique, as well as show how to make transitions at certain points. Some cases can be much wordier and longer and much more elaborate and colorful, with many directions, sidetracks, and a larger, more complex picture.

In this case, I left more of the words that the patient actually said, but I did abridge it in parts as well.)

I began by asking her about the kidney stones.

"When did this begin for you?"

"10 years ago – KI stones began.

They've been tested as uric acid and calcium."

"Which side?"

"Both sides. Cannot say left was more than the right. It was just about equal."

"How does it feel?" (Looks like I jumped in rather quickly with that question in this case. I could have investigated more before diving in with that question. It did work out alright in the end.)

"Pain – it starts out just kind of a little backache – you think 'maybe I turned wrong or something.' And then all of a sudden – it doesn't feel comfortable sitting here. I am going to get up and walk around. It wouldn't hurt as much and then I couldn't sit down anymore. There were a couple of times, it was just out of control. I just waited too long. It just hurts awful. It feels so heavy and is so painful. I cannot stand to sit or stand. There's no comfortable position. I try to walk around, that is the least painful."

"Tell me what the pain feels like?"

"It feels like squeezing. Someone is squeezing my sides.

Feels like someone has got a hold of my sides and is pressure squeezing."

Now this is very interesting because she says *"Someone* is squeezing my sides. Feels like *someone* has got a hold of my sides and is pressure squeezing." So here is an indication that there is a larger picture. It's like a keyhole to a deeper issue has been revealed and we've now managed to take a peek into a larger space.

At this point, we have an invitation to open up the questions toward a larger picture, in terms of the life. I could have asked, at this point, *"Someone is squeezing your sides? Is there anyone that comes to mind that you feel it could be?"*

That is a bit of a jump. It's asking a patient to be very, very mindful *already* about their problem. This doesn't always happen. A smoother, slower transition is usually more effective at establishing a clear connection. It's like allowing Nature to expose the connection organically.

So I continued to dialogue with her about her condition.

"Is there anywhere else in your life where you feel this way – squeezed?"

"Not really. Nothing I can think of."

"What were you doing in your life at the time the kidney stones began 10 years ago? Anything out of the ordinary."

"Nothing special, really. I was working in management as a nurse."

"What was your job like for you?"

"Extremely stressful."

"Tell me about that."

"The job of manager as a nurse was a very difficult position. We had been through so many nurse managers... because it was so stressful. One was crying – she was thrown to the wolves.

I was very competitive so I said, I was going to last the longest."

"What's the stress about in that position?"

"I like to have flowers around me. I like to have things to be calm. I like to be nice to people. In my other world before management – people could walk all over me. When I went into management – that part of me left. I went more into a tougher role because I had to defend the staff from upper management. I took on the position – 'No one is going to run over me.'

I had to develop something other than a passive role.

But then I also had to discipline people, which was very hard for me. The first time I had to discipline someone – it gave me diarrhoea and I felt terrible. I thought they are going to hate me

– if I told them, they are going to hate me."

"What was that like for you?"

"It is the sandwich effect.

Squeezing from both directions."

She said this very spontaneously and at this point, she took a sharp intake of breath and had a huge, beaming smile on her face. I gave this some time for her to marvel at the connection. She used the same expression for the pain in her kidneys. Being *squeezed*. This is at the heart of her stress at work. She is forced into a situation where she has to defend her nurses that she manages from upper management, and also, discipline them at the same time. This makes her feel squeezed. She sat there reflecting about this a little longer and then said:

"I am still being squeezed. Intuitively and consciously tired of the management. I know I am a good manager – I treat my people with respect. I don't see that in a lot of other managers. Nor at homecare or hospital. I am confident in my management role – I have no doubt I am a good manager. But it does take a toll on me. I don't know how to have fun anymore. It is a heavy role. Cannot goof around anymore. I cannot even horse around with these people. (Upper management.) It has taken a huge toll. I am not nice always. I am nice at work – not always so nice to my husband. (O – A lot of weeping here. There is a lot of sadness.) I feel horrible. Sometimes I wonder what it would be like to wake up in the morning and not have that burden. I have had it for so long. I would be so light. You couldn't pull me off the ceiling."

So this case continued to evolve and deepen from this point. The connection between the kidneys feeling squeezed and heavy pain and the squeezing and heavy role as a manager was a great mind-body connection. When she recognized this, it really helped her see how unhealthy a position she was put in for all those years and eventually left her job, which was something she had thought of for a long time. People had been telling her for years to quit her job, but she could not find the courage to do so.

After leaving her job, she began to feel much better and after two more bouts of kidney stones, she no longer had any more kidney stone attacks.

Next Case: *48 year old woman with some form of neurological condition thought to be myasthenia gravis.*
A little background for this case. She has four siblings. Two of her brothers have died. She has difficult relationships with her other two siblings, and they barely speak with each other. She was diagnosed with myasthenia gravis, but there is something else going on with her. The doctors are not sure what it is.

She said: "When it first started, it was so unusual for me. I began writing a diary for it, so the doctors could have the information. History of seeing many doctors. Unusual. The way it came on – suddenly and they couldn't figure out what was causing all these different issues. Several are in agreement that it is a neurological issue. I do have myasthenia gravis, but some of the symptoms have not jived with that. So I am not being treated for that."

She also has several physical complaints with her condition. Including sinus infections. Teeth problems. Heaviness of the limbs. She has periods where she could barely walk. She was placed on many different drugs. Nothing helped. At the time of the appointment, she was on 900 mgs per day of Neurontin, an anti-epileptic, and had been up to 2400 mgs per day when she couldn't walk.

I begin exploring some of the physical symptoms, after she has discussed quite a lot about her family situation with me.
"Tell me about the sinuses."
"Sinuses. Yeah. I just feel tired and that drainage constantly is no fun. But it is not debilitating."
"Where do you feel it?"
"It is at a very deep part of my sinuses. Like deep inside there."

"Anything make it better or worse?"

"Doing Neti pots don't help. It's too deep. I've tried other things. Nothing much helps. It is worse in the evenings."

"Does it stop you from doing anything?"

"Well, I am still working out. I am walking. But my energy level is not where it used to be."

"How do the sinuses feel in there?"

"It's like a weight is pressing. Like a pressure as of a weight in the sinuses."

(At this point she spontaneously began speaking about her teeth.)

"My teeth hurt sometimes. My top teeth ache. The front teeth (4-5 teeth). The ache – it is a dull ache, not sharp, that is always there. It feels like there is a weight weighing on my teeth. A weight is there – I am constantly feeling that weight on my mouth, on my teeth."

At this point, the theme of a weight pressing down became apparent between the two body parts. This is called a *generality* in homeopathy. It's not just in one location; it's now in more than one location.

So I ask: *"Is there anywhere else you feel a weight?"*

"I feel a weight on my legs."

"Where on your legs do you feel it?"

"Right in the top area of the thighs, where they meet my hips."

"What does the weight feel like there?"

"It's heavy. Weighing down. Like I am not able to walk and do what I need to do with that weight there."

"How long have you had that feeling in your legs?"

"It's basically the feeling I've always had that makes it very hard for me to walk. I can't walk or move around well because there is a weight sitting on my legs."

"What does the weight feel like, that is sitting on the top of your legs?"

"It is like someone sitting on my legs."

(Aha! Here is a description of a sensation that points away from just speaking about the body to something outside of the physical. It's a keyhole into a larger picture. So I ask, quite directly, which results in a great response):

"*Who is the 'someone' sitting on your legs?*"

"There is a list of the people sitting on my legs. My husband, my daughter, my family..."

(Earlier, she had spoken a lot about how she felt responsible for everyone, to make sure everyone was happy. With the death of her two brothers, it had really affected the family, and she felt responsible to hold things together, to prevent them from breaking down even further. This puts what comes up next into a clearer context.)

"*Tell me more.*"

"Feels like someone is sitting on my lap all the time. They are nursing on me still. That is how it feels. They are keeping me down."

(She begins seeing the larger picture. She gets excited at this point.)

"*What keeps you down?*"

"They have me... (She reflects further to get the right wording for what she is trying to describe.)

By having me focus on them instead of me focusing on me."

"*How do they have you focus on them instead of yourself?*" (I asked this particular question because with the last statement she really made it sound like they were actively having her focus on them. That didn't reveal much about her part in it.)

"I mean, I am so focused on me making them happy, and it is wearing me out. It makes me feel like my legs have weight."

"*Do you want to keep living this way?*"

"No! I don't! And I don't have to. I realize I have been putting so much energy into making sure everyone is happy so that our family wouldn't fall even more apart."

(Here she cries a lot and a lot of the grief from the loss of her two brothers is expressed. There is also a relief. She sees and understands that she has taken it onto herself to hold everyone together by focusing on making them happy. She begins seeing it very differently and a wonderful, spontaneous healing happens.)

"I can feel the lightening. My legs are lightening. And even my sinuses."

It is amazing to witness this sort of healing. It confirms that the heaviness-weighted generality sensation she had was connected to her core problem. Also, when the core problem was released, being grief where she felt responsible for making everyone happy, and had been carrying them, the actual sensation of heaviness and weakness also lifted. This resulted in a true and lasting healing for her. It had really impacted her body. Here is where we have clear evidence of a mind-body connection. This is the ideal result; to witness the result of letting go of the belief and unhealthy behavior having immediate, or eventual, healing response on the body. This keeps the healing real and prevents us from projecting overly positive, "hopeful" thoughts onto a person. If someone contacts the issue at hand and releases it and the physical body does not improve, either quickly or slowly, then we must be honest about that and keep digging deeper, and look for another solution or even deeper, more hidden cause of the problem. We can also look for obstacles to cure that must be removed.

What can also occur is that the health begins to improve with the release of the core issues as they are initially perceived, and the release of the disease ends up helping heal a larger picture. The first dialogue begins the healing process. The life begins to improve. This brings more free flowing availability for The Healing Power of Nature to enter therein and brings more healing to the deeper, more ingrained issues. We have to follow Nature and let Nature speak. In this case, the root cause was addressed and she changed her mind. It resulted in healing of her entire being.

In the follow-up, she said all of her issues had completely improved, except her sinuses. She also said the following:

"There are so many times I forget to take my medication – because now I know what caused my weakness. As long as I continue to address the emotional issues – I realized that I was worth it and I was enough, by myself. I never allowed myself to feel that before. Whenever I feel down, I say to myself, you are enough and you matter. Everything is much lighter, and I feel so much better about myself and my future. It is just one of those things. I am hoping it will stay forever.

If I get heavy, I have to listen to my body – stressed or tired. I just feel so much lighter. I see my husband in a totally different way now. I was really worried for a while. I didn't know if we were going to make it."

Not only did her health improve, so did her relationships, especially with her husband. She was considering leaving that marriage. The "weight" was too much. With her letting go of the weight she was carrying, she was able to let go of her unhealthy part in the process with her husband, and be there in a healthier fashion to work on things together. It resulted in them moving into a happier, healthier space together.

For our second follow-up, I received the following email, as a response to my confirmation email of our up and coming appointment:

"Hi Dr. Moshe: I am feeling fantastic and won't need a follow-up at this time. If anything changes I will e-mail you! Thanks so much for your help."

I had not heard back from her for three years following that, so I wrote and asked her how things were going and she replied, "I am happy to report that my health is the best it has ever been. I ran three half-marathons last year and I know that would not have been possible if I did not learn how to listen to my body and heal myself from the inside out."

In another case, the mind-body connection became very clear in the exact use of language she used for how her body felt and how her life felt. In that case, we can almost call it a "life-body connection." In the end, since our I AM is what we have that keeps us alive, vibrant, healthy, happy, we can say our I AM statement is our "To Be" statement. "To Be" is "To Live." So, where the life is affected so too will the body become affected. The mind and the life become intimately connected at this point, with any distinction only being in regards to the elements a body or a "life" is made up, and not the energetic essence. Dr. Paul Epstein ND has a very good way of describing this. He says, "Our biography becomes our biology." Carolyn Myss has also used this phrase in her healing work. It's so true.

This is a case of a middle-aged woman who had an auto-immune condition, fibromyalgia, chronic fatigue, reflux, constipation, and insomnia. In each and every appointment we had, through Holistic Counseling, we got to the same core belief, regardless of which condition was flaring up at the time. One condition would improve after it flared up and we focused on it, only to give rise to another issue. She was often asking for some relief from the symptoms. "Give me something for the heartburn." Or, "Give me something for the constipation."

During one of our follow-ups, the arthritis was really acting up.

She said: "I can no longer ignore the pain. It is like a rollercoaster."

Since I had already been working with her for some time, I knew her main issue resided with her husband. They were having a lot of issues as a couple and so when I asked,

"How's it going with your husband?"

She said: "I knew you were going to ask that. It's not going well. I've been feeling like I am on a rollercoaster. It's really painful for me being in the relationship and I realized recently that I really cannot ignore this problem any longer."

She really didn't realize what she had said and how it corresponded to *exactly* what she had said about the pain in her joints (particularly, her hands).

So I said: *"Let me read back to you what you just said: 'I've been feeling like I am on a rollercoaster. It's really painful for me being in the relationship and I realized recently that I really cannot ignore this problem any longer.' What does that sound like?"*

And then she realized, "It's what I said about how my hands feel."

Yes. So we discussed this and the implications for her life. She realized that the pain she was feeling emotionally was making her take a good, hard look at her life. She could no longer ignore what was happening. Her body took on the very same pain and the very same signature. She couldn't ignore it any longer. It was like a rollercoaster. Previously, and for a long time, she had been going to many practitioners, including other naturopaths, just to bring comfort to her symptoms so that she could go on living being in denial of her feelings regarding the situation with her husband. Hers was always an obstinate case and I believe it is for this very reason; that she had not yet dealt with the root of her problem, either by doing what she needed to do to heal her marriage so she could live happily with her husband, or by leaving the relationship. Instead, she lived in a kind of limbo, where her unhappiness, and the underlying core issues she was not dealing with, which was "feeling not good enough", continued to manifest as a multitude of physical symptoms and conditions, all for which she went to doctors, naturopaths, acupuncturists, chiropractors, massage therapists, and osteopaths, to take care of her symptoms. It was no different with me. Despite having helped her recognize the root of her conditions during every appointment, which resulted in some healing of the present condition, the next follow-up, she would have another complaint that was flaring up. I would Holistically

Counsel her and we would arrive, again, at the core of her beliefs. Yet each time, during the beginning of the appointment, she would state all the things she had been doing (doctor appointments, acupuncture) and taking (supplements, drugs, etc.) and complain about the condition that was flaring up as if she still wanted me to give her something that would take away the pain. This is important to recognize as a Holistic practitioner. Helping a person see the mind-body connection does not mean they are going to immediately get with the program and be forever changed. Sometimes they do quickly. Sometimes moderately quickly. Sometimes slow. And sometimes it is a very difficult, stuck situation that takes a lot of time and many repetitions of awareness in order to sink in.

I think it was easy for her to forget because of the great many practitioners she went to that just kept reaffirming the false model of "Here. Take this; it will help you feel better with your *'whatever it is you're struggling with now'* condition." Even when I offered her a homeopathic remedy to assist her in her process of healing her life by changing her beliefs about herself, I could sense a "glossing over" of the eyes and forgetting her own inner work. It was as if that clarity she was experiencing and the resulting empowerment that came from her recognizing her choice in all her conditions, was going out the window when she was offered the "thing" she could hold onto that would do the work for her. That is why I am careful to not offer anything following a really good Holistic Counseling session. I do not want to interfere at all with the profound process of change that is going on in the patient following their awareness of their core belief and the subsequent choice to change that belief. Even giving a homeopathic, I have seen, can alter that clarity. This is what Dr. Paul Epstein calls, "Homeopathy without the remedy."[17]

How on Earth has our world ever gotten to the point where a person prefers to take something rather than become empowered to heal themselves with a change in mind that will have an everlasting positive effect on their lives? The answer is obvious for many of us. The conventional and allopathic model of medicine. Pharmaceutical and now, Nutraceutical, marketing of drugs and supplements. And perhaps most of all, even the so-called alternative medicine and Naturopathic medicine world mostly has been able to offer only the same allopathic solutions. Yes, those solutions are less toxic, more natural, more well-thought out, considered on a more "global" solution (Systems model), but are, nevertheless, ignoring the most important dimension – and that is the life and the mind level and how that connects with the physical dimension of pathology. And this brings me to one of the most important elements about the process of true Holistic healing that I can express. And that is the implications for the soul's Evolution.

Implications for the Evolution of the Soul

Imagine if this patient had been able to receive a successful suppression of her symptoms? Imagine all of the practitioners she had gone to, had been able to keep her conditions from acting up? What would the implication have been for her life, her choices and the evolution of her soul?

When we die, we bring nothing with us that is of this physical world. That all goes down into the ground, or up in smoke, leaving our bodies nothing but ash. I believe the only things we bring are the life lessons that we learn that are learned at a deep enough level to be carried forward into the very fabric of our being. That occurs through our soul. And what better life lessons can we learn than the ones that have been so very challenging for us that they have resulted in actual physical, or mental-emotional disease?

Let's look at the implication of this for the present case. She had been on many supplements and also some pretty heavy-duty drugs, one being Plaquinyl, a serious drug that is normally administered for Malaria, but was given to her for her auto-immune disease. It is a drug that is not recommended to be taken over a long period of time. She had been on it for 20 years. I slowly had her come off the Plaquinyl, along with the other drugs and supplements that kept being offered to her from other practitioners. This is one of the main reasons I wrote the article in the NDNR titled: "Managing Mind-Body Medicine in a World of Obstacles."[18]

Here, the obstacles were the allopathic mindset – everywhere, including with other naturopaths, making it so easy for her to forget to focus on the deepest and most positively influential issues.

What resulted from her coming off all the meds and the supplements came to a head in this last appointment that I just shared, where she stated that the pain in her hands was so much now that *she could no longer ignore it*. I think this case, right at this point, more than anything, really exemplifies the life lesson that kept getting deferred by being able to just quell the conditions with more supplements, more practitioner intervention on the level of the body. By her not being able to just alleviate and ultimately, suppress, the symptoms, she was forced into a choice. She could no longer avoid the issue at hand. And what was that? It wasn't the symptoms of the body she was really speaking about. Those were just the messengers of the expression of her unhappy Vital Force that was being suppressed in a painful situation. The real issue resided within her relationship with her husband. But even that was not the real issue. The real issue for this patient was her core belief that she was not good enough. This belief that came up during every Holistic Counseling session at the root of whatever condition she was struggling with at the present time, was at the root for her making a choice to believe that her unhappy marriage was acceptable because she wasn't good enough to deserve better, to have happiness, health, or her needs met. This core issue was so very deep for her, and so incredibly challenging, that she would rather do everything else besides face it. This is another reason why her case kept "relapsing" into "give me something for the condition doctor."

And the choice was so difficult that it just so happens that it took the kind of pain that makes someone say, "I just cannot ignore this any longer." And that is what she did. She stopped ignoring it and got really tough, recognizing what she deserved as a fundamental need for any relationship, and she made some demands with her husband that represented her boundaries and her being true to herself. She felt she was moving forward in her life (this was one of the physical manifestations also of her symptoms in her articulations – she had the pain in her joints as being "held back," and this also pointed to how she felt in her life, for obvious reasons). Her symptoms dramatically improved while she remained strong and true to herself. Later, again, she had a bit of a relapse, although not as severe as her symptoms had been, when she began to doubt herself, and got stuck in worrying about her husband's well-being and again not being balanced with her own well-being. Yet, having had that experience of strength and dedication to what was important for her, along with the improvement of her condition, it provided her a beacon to follow in the future to reclaim her strength, which resulted in improvement of her health.

Would she have faced this most difficult choice if she had continued on all the drugs and supplements that just kept the symptoms from pressing her into change? Would she have grown through the challenge of her life's lesson?

The answer is I believe she would not have faced this most difficult choice for her. Or, she may have waited a long time until she had some even worse health crisis due to all the suppression of the expression of her symptoms. That may have brought some awakening. But it also may have been too late to be able to embark on the path of healing without heroic allopathic measures.

In our lives, our symptoms are caused by making choices that are misaligned and untrue for us. This error in choice, sometimes innocently, but nevertheless at our own hands leads to a problem. Does it make any sense to create a problem and then not deal with it at its source? It's like a teenager who continues to make a great mess around the house that is disruptive to the rest of the family. If the parents simply keep cleaning the house up, what message does it impart to the teenager? The implications for the rest of the teenager's life, that is, the evolution of their life is greatly compromised. By just offering a solution to take away a problem that a patient is responsible for creating in their lives, are we not doing the same thing as these parents? Are we not doing some harm? Sure the parents have a soft side for their child but is tough love not a most loving way of being for their child who continues to make the same mistake?

It just so happens that Nature does force us toward healing even if we're on tons of drugs. The drugs stop working. They really do, because they offer no lasting solution. The need for the expression of the Vital Force's mistunement is so strong, that it usually does find a way of becoming expressed even in the face of great opposition and suppression. And if by some chance, the drugs and/or supplements are strong enough to keep all expressions of the out of tune Vital Force from surfacing that is a great and most serious tragedy. We might as well straightjacket the soul while we're at it.

As practitioners we cannot make the change that a patient needs to make. We can lead them to water, through the Vis Dialogue, but we cannot make them drink. If and when they drink is a choice that is theirs to make. Hopefully, for their sake, they make it in a timely, expedient fashion. But if not, there is nothing we can do except hold the awareness of what is the best direction for them to take and lead them back to water during subsequent appointments.

The awareness of what a person's problem is can be revealed

by the patient. It emerges from the patient and not from a projection of the practitioner. We are there to encourage them to make the choice. We should never lose sight of where their soul's evolution is calling them to go, even if they do. The importance of this will become clear to the practitioner when they deal with long, protracted cases where they have to act as the "Lighthouse" to keep the patients coming back to the source of the problem. I say this also because it can be easy to give up on someone. I admit that I have felt the inclination to do so on several occasions with patients who get all wrapped up in allopathic suppression following our deep diving sessions together. It can be greatly frustrating to see a patient walk away from their healing Truth. Yet, I remind myself what I am there for. I reset the intention to help them and to be in my heart, for their highest good. And then, in the beginning of that next appointment, after hearing them describe to me what their doctors or other healthcare practitioners have given them to help them with their condition, I take a deep internal breath and dive back into the questions with them. At first, I have to overcome the inertia of the allopathic boulder that has rolled back onto them. And I really am amazed at how deeply we can go, despite their doubt, despite their propensity for seeking suppressive therapies. We always go deep. Sometimes the best follow-ups are following these sorts of departures from the Holistic path.

I do find it baffling how quickly patients say, "It's not working." Despite having very clear and excellent improvements using mind-body medicine, when they relapse, or the symptoms return, some patients so easily wave a hand and dismiss the healing and say that it doesn't work. This was true in this case, and in many other cases that are a little up and down, though with a general upward trend. There will be an improvement. They will feel better than they have, sometimes ever, and sometimes for a long time. Nothing else has even touched their condition and they have seen improvement by applying the changes that we brought forth in the mind-body medicine. And even so, even with the improvements, they will quickly, almost snappishly claim, "It's not working," if there's any sort of relapse. These patients do not want to relinquish the mindset that they have no say in their health. They want to quickly look outside for a reason to blame for their health concerns. And what better thing to blame than the medicine for not working. I pray this tendency will change for patients to want to give away their self-empowering responsibility over their health. I know that with time and as more and more practitioners help guide patients toward the Truth about how The Healing Power of Nature works inside of them in a Holistic, mind-body sense, this will gain an accelerated shift out of medicine's dark ages.

Yet for the time being, because the dark ages still have a hold and appeal over much of the masses, as a practitioner, I know I have to commit to being the "Lighthouse." I have chosen to never be a practitioner that just alleviates symptoms, because those symptoms are a message from the deeper part of the patient to be heard.

Balancing the Idealism: What I have written in this book is true, in accordance with the knowledge I have come to understand about healing at this point in time. Having said that, the world is not an ideal place, and so, even though medicine may be applied in great alignment with the ideal form of healing, it may not always result in the kind of healing we'd like to see. There are times when we have to treat allopathically to save a patient's life, or temporarily alleviate their suffering, and in Chapter 36 on "The Limitations of Holistic Counseling" I discuss this further. Also, in other times, a patient is so overwhelmed by their symptoms, they cannot use their mind to make choices to heal. They need some relief. That is not a sin. It would be an error of idealism to refuse to do anything that is allopathic in cases where it is called for. It is rare that the allopathic approach does need to be the case, but when it is called for, if one refuses to act allopathically, then one has allowed Holistic healing to become a religious dogma, and we all know where that leads. But in the great majority of the time, in my practice, I do not have to resort to allopathic symptomatic relief, and can remain aligned with the principles of Holism that I know will result in the greatest healing and implications for the person's life and soul's purpose and evolution.

However, we, as practitioners, must not make the error of being overly idealistic when a simple solution can stave off a patient's suffering for enough time for them to regain composure in life and then dive back into their deeper healing. This is a bit of a gray area, and depends on the discretion of the practitioner, because sometimes a case appears to need allopathic help but in the end, can be resolved through Holism alone. And other times, a person is so depressed and lacking energy that they cannot function. They cannot change their mindset. They are paralyzed emotionally. They are "caught in the tentacles of the octopus." Then, they need a little boost. It can even be for a short time, and that is all they needed to get back on their feet, ready for the healing. Just remember that a practitioner that can heal a case holistically is offering a much greater service than if they treat allopathically, where it is not necessary.

Do not forget the simple obstacles to cure. A patient is drinking toxic water. They are living 100 meters from a cellphone tower or an electrical plant. They have mercury amalgams that are leaching mercury into their bodies. They have an underlying infection that is not fully resolving with the mind-body medicine and keeps returning any time the patient is under any stress. Whatever the case may be, I present the vision of medicine in its ideal and most true form, to correct the great misuse of allopathic medicine that has come to take over this planet. However, it is for the practitioner to keep their mind open to times when the allopathic approach, or the removal of the obstacles to cure, is the right approach.

The way a person feels about their illness & what it makes them do or not do is often an indication of what led to the illness in the first place.

In the last case, we saw that the patient felt that she couldn't ignore the pain in her hands. This was a reflection of the fact that she couldn't ignore the painful situation in her life. In the earlier case about the woman with multiple sclerosis, when exploring how she felt about her illness, she said she felt trapped because she couldn't leave her house. Upon further exploration, her illness was a manifestation of a chronic state of her mother forcing herself on the patient and the patient feeling trapped, like there was nothing she could do.

I had a case of myasthenia gravis of a man in his sixties that responded very well to the homeopathic remedy Corvus-corax. He was basically symptom free, until one day, he called me and said he was having a relapse of his symptoms. He said he was so weak and he couldn't leave his house to come and see me. He asked if I could come to see him at his house. This was interesting because it turned out to be a reflection of what caused his relapse. The story was that, as is seen in some of the bird remedies, homeopathically, in particular Eagle (Halieetus leucocephalus) and Raven (Corvus corax), in addition to there being a need for freedom, both these remedies derive a lot of pleasure from driving fast. They have a need for speed. So did my patient. In fact, he loved driving fast so much that he had amassed quite a few speeding tickets that he decided he wasn't going to pay. The government took away his license. It was a shock to him and upset him very much. He said, "I feel trapped in my apartment. I cannot leave without my license. The thing I love most has been taken away from me. I am stuck in the apartment." So the very thing that he was feeling about his condition, "trapped" and what his condition forced upon him, "I can't leave" was a direct reflection of what had brought on the relapse of the myasthenia gravis.

In another case of a man in his forties with Polymyositis, when he would describe how he felt with the condition, he said that he couldn't stand up very straight. His body felt so weak that he couldn't stand up. Upon exploration of his life in general, he had an issue with one of his brothers that he partnered with for their family business. His brother had a very strong, imposing personality. My patient did not feel comfortable confronting his brother and would not stand up to him. So over time, with enough of the emotion suppressed, with enough of "not standing up," his illness eventually manifested into the very situation that had led to it – he could not stand up.

So two questions help bring up this connection between how the illness feels and what led to it.

"How does the illness feel?" Literally, how does it feel?

And:

"How do you feel about the illness?" It's like asking, *"How do you feel about the fact that you have the illness?"* Or, *"How do you feel since you have the illness?"*

Another question that is relevant is, *"What does the illness stop you from doing?"*

Example: "I can't take care of myself now that I have the illness." Upon closer examination, cases that have this can very likely also have the very issue of not taking care of themselves as their history, even before the disease manifested. Or, we can say that a person has always been taken care of, most likely, by their parents, and due to some circumstance, perhaps natural growing up, maturing and leaving the house, or by some tragedy, they are no longer in a situation where the parents can take care of them. The reaction, at this point, can be to state to oneself, "I don't want to take care of myself" albeit in a more subconscious and less overtly expressed and understood fashion. Such a strong statement and desire, to not want to take care of oneself, can lead to an illness where a person is unable to take care of themselves.

I have not seen this direct correlation between the cause of the illness and the actual expression about the illness by the patient in every case. However, it happens often enough that it is unmistakeable and quite inspiring to witness when it does occur.

The Way a Patient feels about their Drugs is a Reflection of the Patient's Wound/Need

This is similar to the previous topic, yet with a different twist. It is related to how people feel about their drugs. Both coming off them and also how they feel when they are on them.

People go on or reach for drugs in order to suppress their symptoms. That is plain and simple. So the fears that they feel about coming off their drugs relates entirely to what they feel will rise up once they stop the drugs. Even more importantly, the reason the person feels they need the drug is a direct reflection of what they fear they lack inside of themselves. So the drugs become little helpers that reflect a person's need or fear.

For example, in one case, a woman was very used to suppressing her feelings. It was a way of life for her. So when she got very depressed from suppressing her feelings, she is then put on a drug that continues that same suppression she is already doing to herself. In another example, one I have seen in many cases, a person feels that they lack support. Their parents or partners don't support them, so they reach for their drug or supplements as a means of filling the void of the lack of support. It can really be any form of drug. It doesn't matter so long as the patient feels supported by it. In another example that reveals a slightly different angle on this topic, a patient had a sense of slipping into darkness at different points of her life. When she was there, I asked her what she looked to in order to get herself out. She said she felt like there was a rope that she could grab onto to pull her out of the darkness. She could only do so sometimes. Later, when we discussed her coming off the Lexapro, she expressed a fear that she won't have any rope to pull her out of the darkness. So for her, the drug does take on the role of helper in the very same way the person feels they lack inside themselves. This is expressed uniquely in every case.

So the drug can be both a reflection of what a person already does to themselves – suppresses themselves. Or it can be a means of filling a void. Lacking support. Needing a rope out of darkness. It takes on the nature of the patient's fear and suppression. We can learn a lot about how a patient really feels underneath the drug they're on, depending on how suppressed their feelings are, when we begin to discuss coming off the drug. And it should be so. Because as they come off it, they are faced only with themselves and what has been suppressed by the drug, or the lack that they feel in themselves for which they relied on the drug.

The Metaphor of the Two Cabooses – The Momentum of Illness in the Body

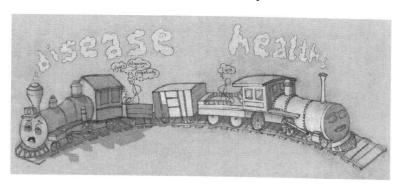

Here is another metaphor that can be helpful during different appointments to explain to a patient what is occurring for them in regards to their health, and what might occur with their physical condition in the near future.

Imagine a train with a caboose at each end that point in opposite directions. One is the Caboose of health and the other is the Caboose of disease. Unfortunately, when someone is sick, they have been shoveling a lot of coal into the Caboose of disease. So much so, that the train has gained quite a lot of momentum in the direction of the disease. This can be seen in the physical body where a patient has been "shoveling" so much fuel into the negative beliefs and the subsequent control that has been affected on the Three Treasures mind-Qi-blood cascade that the disease seems to have a mind of its own. The disease can be described as something very much separated from the patient, like it is a living, breathing entity with a life of its own. At this point, a patient will express that their symptoms come on for "no apparent reason." (There is always a reason, but it may be beyond the patient's awareness.)

I have seen cases where the root cause of the disease was addressed and even removed, only to have symptoms continue to act out in the body. Here the *Metaphor of the Two Cabooses* is of great importance. As the patient had continued to shovel fuel into the Caboose of disease, their train has gathered a lot of momentum in the direction of the disease. Even when the person stops shoveling coal into the engine, the disease can live on for some time. It's due to the "momentum" it has gathered from the past. I witnessed this in the case of the woman with kidney stones. She resolved the core issue and began to really heal and move in the right direction of healing, but there was still some momentum of the disease on the physical plane. So even after she resolved the source of her problem, she still had another couple of bouts of kidney stones. Once these had "exhausted the momentum" of disease in the physical body, she no longer had any more pain, nor any attacks of kidney stones.

The physical body, being quite dense in nature, responds slower than the higher worlds of the emotion, mind, and Spirit/soul. It is still a reflection of them, but the effect of a thought on the emotions can be immediate, whereas, it can take time to reach the body. The "time lag" between the physical and mental-emotional realms varies from person to person. For some sensitive people, they can have a thought that is not healthy for them and then have to run immediately to the toilet. A sensitive person has a physical body that responds quickly, like the strong winds in the sails of a small, light ship. Any small unharmonious thought can result in a fast mirrored reaction in the body. Worried thinking can quickly bring on a headache. Resisting unpleasant feelings can bring on a tightening of muscles right away. I've seen cases of myasthenia gravis go from very weak and sick, to feeling very healthy and strong with the switch of their core beliefs, only to return to weakness when those original false thoughts are "reshoveled" into the firebox of their Caboose of disease.

I also think that the amount of lag between the body and mind has to do with the amount of healing a person has gone through and done on themselves. People who eat well, meditate, work on their issues, experience a lot of healing, and have opened their mind to a picture that is beyond the parameters of the world limited to the physical, tend to have a physical body that is higher in vibrational frequency than a person who lives unaware of the greater mysteries of this world. Such a highly tuned body normally responds faster to Holistic/mind-body healing.

The factors affecting "time lag" between mental shoveling and body response is probably quite a complex picture since a person can have worked on themselves, but came into life with an already very dense body. Or a person is very sensitive and has next to no lag without having done any previous healing. I imagine the distribution of the elements in their astrological birth chart plays a role, with energies like earth and water signs and planets predisposing a person more toward a dense and slower responding body. It would also depend on where those signs and planets were placed. The amount of lag time between the healing of the root cause in the mental-emotional sphere and the body catching up in the healing also depends on how long a person has been sick and which organs or parts of the body are affected. Brain pathologies, for instance, can take longer time to respond to healing, whereas the rest of the nervous system can have more rapid changes. A person who has been sick for a long time can also take longer to see results at the physical level simply due to how invested they are into the reality of their illness from their long history with it. It's like they've gotten used to the sick reality, and cannot even fathom that they could be well. This will progress slowly.

Suffice it to say that there is a lag between the body and the mind and it varies from person to person and between conditions. Interestingly enough, there is also a lag between the mind and emotions. People will often declare that they grasp something intellectually, but they *feel* differently. So they understand the belief and they want to let it go, but they don't feel like they can. The mind, relative to the emotions, is masculine, whilst the emotions are feminine. The mind decides upon something (*Agens*) and the emotions take on the nature of the belief and will reflect this through the sensations of feeling (*Patiens*). Those emotions have a greater level of inertia, since they are "denser" in nature to the mind. So even when a thought shifts or is released, the emotions reacting to the former belief can have some inertia and need to play themselves out.

Here is the crux of the matter. The healing begins right when a patient stops shoveling energy into the firebox of the Caboose of disease. Even if the effects on the body have not been immediately realized, the healing does really begin right with the change of perspective. With a new choice comes new direction. At first, the train may still maintain a lot of momentum toward disease, but in time, it will first slow down and eventually stop moving in the direction of disease. At this point, the disease will stop affecting the body and then the train can begin to gain momentum in the direction of the reversal of disease and health.

Imagine the meddlesome nuisance of conventional medicine and the allopathic model at the point where a person has already begun healing, but they insist on continuing to take allopathic medicines or supplements. These suppress the expression of the symptoms and ultimately cause the train to be pushed again by the Caboose of disease. The beginning of healing can be a very delicate time, as in when a flower is first unfolding from its bud. The allopathic model can stop any momentum of the healing process dead in its tracks and push the momentum back toward the direction of disease.

Trust is such an important mindset in the business of Holistic healing because of the momentum an illness can have even following the dissolution of its root cause. There are times when I know I need to explain this to patients so they have the patience to wait out the change of momentum of their illness, and to trust that, with the root cause of their disease removed, The Healing Power of Nature can enter into the picture and do its wonders. And, like so many other things in Nature, its healing power can take time.

I also explain to patients that they will probably continue to think the unhealthy thoughts from time to time that led to their illness. It's pretty normal. This shovels a little more fuel into the firebox of the Caboose of disease, and there can be a little back and forth in the first days and weeks of healing. But because the engine of the Caboose of healing is already fired up and has begun to push toward the direction of healing, the 'slips' toward disease harbour less momentum and are easier to recover from. Patients will express this by saying things like; "I got a migraine again, but it wasn't as bad and didn't last as long." Or, "I felt depressed again yesterday, but it wasn't as severe. Even though I felt so depressed, I also knew I was ok at the same time, like I had some choice within it. I could pull myself out of it much easier." That is the momentum of healing speaking, and despite the ever-abating yet-still-present momentum of disease, the patient knows they are getting better. If they forget, you can share with them this metaphor of the *Two Cabooses*.

Chronic Effects of Physical Injury and the Underlying Cause

When a person has a physical injury that is not healing very well over time, it is important to take into account the surrounding situation that was present during the time of the injury, in a very similar way to how one takes a history surrounding any condition.

"What was happening for you at the time of the injury?"

Of great importance are the questions, *"What did you feel right before or during the injury?"*

Or, *"What was going through your mind right before or at the time of the injury?"*

What I have found is that a physical injury cannot properly heal when the issues on the mental-emotional levels that led to the circumstances surrounding the injury have yet to be addressed and resolved.

One case was of a young woman who had a broken ankle that would not heal properly. She had several surgeries that were not helping. With her, as with any such case, it was important to investigate what was going on during or just prior to the injury. Through investigation with Holistic Counseling, the story that unfolded was as follows: She was hanging out with her boyfriend and his friends. They were jumping off a bridge into a river. She felt the need to impress them and she jumped as well, which resulted in her breaking her leg. It became clear that she was trying to impress her boyfriend and his friends because she needed to do so in order to compensate for her feeling that she wasn't lovable. And this pattern of working hard and doing things to impress others to compensate for her feeling unlovable was still going on following the injury to her ankle. She was doing so at work, and with her friends, exhausting herself because she was still trying hard to impress others. So the ankle could not heal while the very reason for the original injury to it was still being perpetrated.

When I was in my clinical year at CCNM in 1999, there was a case that another clinician had of a woman who had been paralyzed from the waist down for over 10 years. The history of her case was that she had been in an abusive marriage. She decided she could no longer handle it and told her husband that she wanted to end the relationship. She did so while they were up on the second-floor balcony. He pushed her off the balcony and she fell and injured her spine in the lumbar area, resulting in her paralysis and inability to walk or move her lower limbs. It was only when she began talking about the trauma and dealing with her emotions regarding the whole situation of her past that she began to heal and regain the use of her legs.

During one of my Holistic Counseling courses, a fascinating case emerged that was the demonstration of the Holistic Counseling technique in front of the class. The gist of the case was that this woman had a terrible injury while she was biking. She had been biking fast and had hit something in her way, flew off her bike and was flying through the air, knowing she was about to impact the side of a truck. Through the dialogue, the following pattern became revealed: what the injury caused her to do was to withdraw from life. Remember, this is a tell-tale sign that is related to the cause. What a condition makes a person do is related to what caused it. I asked her what she did right before the impact. She said that she withdrew her consciousness and blanked out, even before impact. It was as if she wasn't there right at the time of impact. I asked her when this pattern began – after the injury or before? Was there a precedent for this withdrawing from life pattern? She said she had been doing it since she was a child. She did not feel that her parents really listened to her or had created a family environment that was good for her. They were very intellectual types and she was creative and emotional. So, feeling unsupported and not under-stood, she had learned to withdraw into her own world. There were many things in life she had a hard time dealing with. Her response was to withdraw. This thread, therefore, became very impactful in the understanding of her injury that she had not recovered from. Her tendency to withdraw occurred even right before impact, as if the injury was forcing her to face and deal with her choice to withdraw from life and reality. With such a situation, the challenge and difficulty of the lessons get amplified tenfold, as it did for her. She recognized this choice to withdraw and when I began offering her some *Closing questions*, like, *"Do you want to keep living this way?"* she finally decided to choose a new way for herself, her breathing opened up and she felt a sense of peace and healing return to her body.

I've noticed that one of the reasons someone gets injured by accident is that they are not being present in a situation that calls for total presence. Interestingly, what is going through their minds at the time of the injury, that is keeping them from being mindful and aware of dangers or risks around them, is usually some form or permutation of their core issue that they are focusing on instead of being present in the moment. I once witnessed an injury at a healing retreat in Michigan that I taught at that exemplified this. At the gathering on the final day, there were many acknowledgments being offered for those who had done a lot of work to facilitate the retreat. When one of the teenage boys was called down to accept a thank-you gift, I could see he was not being present. He seemed very preoccupied and uncomfortable with the attention. Sure enough, he tripped on one of the stairs and badly sprained his ankle. Later, as he lay on a table nursing his injured ankle, I asked him what was going through his mind right before he hurt himself. He told me he felt embarrassed and didn't like being the center of attention. He was trying to "hide inside of himself." His issue around being the center of attention, which is something that could be explored with Holistic Counseling, was occupying his mind at the time of the injury. And this is another way of seeing disease and injury. It is because something occupies a person which is like a foreign invader that displaces the healthy living presence of a person inside their body, centered in the moment. The injury to the body will not be able to heal so long as that which displaced or "invaded" or was *allowed to invade* the person at and before the time of injury is acknowledged, dealt with and released.

Chapter 31

Closing Questions and Closing Situations

"Do you want to keep living that way?"
"Is this how you want to be?"
"Is this who you really are?"
"What's stopping you from letting that go?"
"What's stopping you from changing that idea or pattern?"
"Are you ready to let that go?"
"Are you going to let that go?"
"Can you let that go?"
"What will you do now?"
"How is that going to look?"
"How are you going to live from now on?"

Ok. We've worked hard with the patient and exposed a belief system, a way of thinking, and a pattern of behavior that seems to be lying as the foundation of their House of Cards. The belief is negative. It's limiting. It's causing stress, unhappiness, suffering, and illness. It is not in harmony with their true I AM statement. It's the last thing you arrived at after a series of questions following the stream. You were asking all these questions to get *somewhere*, and the belief *is* the somewhere that you've arrived at. Now it's time to ask some of the *Closing questions*.

The primary purpose of asking the *Closing questions* is to get the patient to make a declaration of change. You want them to say, "No. I don't want to keep living this way. And yes, I am ready to change." And most importantly, "Yes. I am going to change." Then you dialogue with them about the kind of change they will make. You can devise a plan with them, a strategy, discuss journaling, and also how the change might look. We'll look at all of this in more detail later in Chapter 33 on homework.

In the most basic sense, what a closing situation is really doing is getting a patient to reflect on, *"Is this how you want to be?"* Remember, I AM is from the verb to Be. So the Closing question is really asking a patient, *"Is this who you really are?"*

People can get very, very close to making a change without making a change. They will hesitate, hem and haw, make excuses, change the topic, start telling stories, make a break for it. This is all an attempt to negate setting into motion change that will set them free and result in the death of the ego and the illness, both that are closely connected together and that vie for survival by resisting the change. So as a practitioner, we cannot let the ego and the illness win by allowing it to get away with sabotaging the change or by circumventing the final choice to decide to make a change. It is true that a person can say they are going to make a change and not really follow through with it. But I have found that is less of a problem than a person getting close to making a change and actually not making any sort of declaration for change. Then they have an excuse, an easy way out. They never said they were going to change their beliefs. They never said it, so they don't have to make a change. And thus, nothing has changed. It is true that the awareness of what has been uncovered is healing in and of itself. Like fungus, the dark thoughts of the subconscious cannot exist as much when they are revealed into the light. And so with some patients, possibly, even if they do not commit, they can have some positive effects of having the belief revealed in the earlier part of the Vis Dialogue. But the push to commit usually makes a big difference.

Herein lies a subtlety of the healing. We do not push our awareness on the patient. We do not try to control the outcome of the healing stream of their consciousness. But when it comes down to the wire, when the patient has recognized that the belief is actually not helping them in the way they thought it was, and that they no longer wish to live that way, and we notice that they are faltering, hesitating, backtracking, etc., then we can continue to "press on" with the questions. Or as they try to "get up and flee," we gently bring them back to their center and ask them the questions again. Now, this does not mean that we are forcing them. It means we will keep bringing back the questions along with the feedback necessary to help make the change. If, after several unsuccessful attempts to help the patient declare a new way of seeing things results in continual stuckness, then we will have to change gears. There is also Chapter 32 I have written to address what to do when the case is not advancing or is stuck.

Transition (into Closing) Questions

Transition questions come right before *Closing questions*. I am sharing this topic here, because the topics overlap and it is helpful to share them together. The point of the *Transition question* is to help the patient go from seeing their core belief as their saviour, as something positive, as a means of survival, into recognizing it as something negative and that it is actually not serving them. Because of the candy they think their beliefs reward them with, and because of the compensation as part of the second path, their belief and negative behavior can have the *appearance* of being good for them. So these questions help the patient to separate themselves from the positive attachments to the beliefs and allow them to see them for the negative impact they have on their nature that the beliefs truly are. Then, it becomes clear that they are worthy of release and we can move into the *Closing questions*.

"How's that working out for you?" is a *Transition question*. Often, people think their belief is serving them. It's what they want. One woman had an issue of not having a voice and feeling very angry and frustrated about it. The Vis Dialogue we did together brought her all the way back to the womb, where she had a strong feeling of being forced by Pitocin into induced labour before she was ready. This made her extremely angry and frustrated. This theme of being forced carried itself forward into

her life where she felt like she had no voice to counteract things that she felt forced her against her will. The belief that had been embedded deeply inside her mind, which is a very creative child-like perspective, was that her voice was the actual anger and the frustration. That gave her a voice. She clung onto that as her actual voice. This was all happening deeply on a subconscious level. When I asked her if she ever expressed this anger at all to anyone, she said that she didn't. So I asked her if the expression was internalized, and she said, "Yes." So, I gave her some feedback.

"So, the voice you have is one of anger and frustration that is not actually expressed at all. It's internalized. Is that correct?" She said, "Yes." Then I asked, *"Is that working for you as a voice?"*

This is a spin-off of the same type of Transition question, *"How's that working out for you?"* She said it wasn't. This was quite different from what she had said earlier, because she was very invested in the anger and didn't seem to want to let go of it. The reason she didn't want to let go of the anger became clear. Because she believed it was her voice and it was serving her. But upon actual investigation, it then also became clear that if that is her actual voice, it is not doing what she wants it to be doing – actually speaking up for her or giving her a voice. And that is the point of the *Transition questions* – to disinvest and detach from the connection to a false or negative belief system.

Then I asked her, *"Do you want to keep living that way?"* That is a *Closing question*. Finally, she said, "No." Even going from, "I want to keep living this way. This is good for me." to, "No, I don't want to." is a big step. Depending on the patient, some can take this and run with it, because they have recognized that this is not how they want to live any longer.

I know a patient has already begun healing when they begin stating things that are opposite of what they had claimed earlier. For example, I often hear people say that nobody likes them.

They feel despised. Later, by exploring these beliefs and thoughts and *choices*, they begin spontaneously speaking about people that actually do like them. It's as if a cloud has parted and they can see the light, whereas before, it was a blanket statement of negativity that covered their entire perception of their life. We saw this in the case of the woman with severe eczema, who said her parents didn't love her change her expression to say that she knew her parents loved her. I've also seen this in cases of people that claim they are incapable, or everything will fall apart and fail, as they say it always does. As we continue to explore together, and they begin to see through the absoluteness of their belief, they begin to state new things like, "I can do that. That's really not that much of a problem for me." As is often the case regarding matters of the mind and consciousness, they may not even recognize the stark difference in their attitude and view of things from just a matter of minutes earlier. This is seen a lot in homeopathy with remedies that change people in subtle ways. They don't notice it or even attribute it to either the homeopathy or the counseling. I will point this out to them so that they can see how a little change of mind brings a big change in attitude. Then they can see. What matters most is that the change is already occurring.

"What are you getting out of believing that?"
"How does it serve you?"

These are two more *Transition questions* that we can ask to help shift from "This is good for me and I want to believe it," to "This is not good for me. I no longer want it." These questions are asking someone to seek a positive answer from within a mindset that most likely is strictly limiting and negative. So the ideal answer at this point would be, "I guess I am really not getting anything out of it. It doesn't serve me at all."

However, if a person finds some way of continuing to justify a belief, or if they begin justifying the compensation they are doing to run from their fears, then follow the stream from that point and ask the next pertinent regular questions. Or if it is called for, ask another *Transition question* that is most appropriate.

For example, a person with a lot of anxiety and stress around speaking with colleagues and peers at work states: "I need to make sure I never make any mistakes when I speak with others at work."

"How does that serve you?"

"It makes certain that others will respect me."

"What if others did not respect you?" or we could ask, *"What makes you need others to respect you?"* There is a connection made in asking *"What makes you need others to serve you?"* It's like a feedback because it has a slight additional element added. It is making a connection between the first statement, "I need to make sure" and then them saying, "It makes certain that others will respect me." So to ask, *"What makes you need"* is a fair question without assumption.

Answer: "I need others to respect me so that I can get my work done properly."

Right now, we can see that with *Transition questions*, just as with any other sort of question, including Closing questions, a new avenue may be opened up that is at a deeper place than before. So when this happens, we know that where we thought was the bottom line core belief, is really just another channel in the *Rabbit Hole* or another level in the *House of Cards*. So we keep following the Stream.

"What makes you need others to respect you to get your work done?"

"Without respect, I am unable to work properly."

"What is it about respect that helps you accomplish your work?"

"It feels like what I need in order to be able to concentrate and focus properly on duties."

"What if you don't have respect? What happens when you try to work then?"

"I am missing something."

"What are you missing?"

"I am missing… something. I can't quite put my finger on it."

"Where do you feel like you're missing something?"

Points to his solar plexus area.

"What does it feel like in there?"

"Feels like a void. An emptiness that feels squishy."

"Can you think of any other time or in another situation in your life you may have felt this squishiness?" (That's a *Reflecting Elsewhere question.*)

"Yes. With my father. I used to feel this way with my father. He would only treat me with respect when I got everything right. If I ever made a mistake, he would insult me and criticize me."

"How did that make you feel?"

"Small. Squished. And like he didn't respect me."

"So what did you do when you felt like he didn't respect you?"

"I would try to win back his respect."

"How would you do that?"

"By making sure I got everything perfectly right."

Aha!! This feeds back to the original issue at hand of a person being very anxious that they would lose respect with their colleagues and upper management at work, and as a result, tried to make sure they never said anything wrong. This is a very clear thread that matches completely with the original wound with the father. It is very likely the core issue and the matter at hand at this point. So this is a good clue, an indication that we have arrived at something very core – because the original issue we began consulting about has "folded in back onto itself." Like the beginning and the end line up and mirror each other. This is a Hermetic teaching: "The beginning is in the end and the end is in the beginning." The thread is apparent inside of this, so we know we have touched "ground zero" for the House of Cards.

So here, we can give some feedback about the situation. Or we can just ask a question which calls the original issue to mind.

"Is the way you seek respect by trying not to make mistakes at work the same as the way in which you just said you had to do with your father?"

"Very much so."

"So can we say that as a result of the way your father would respond to you if you made a mistake, you would feel disrespected, small, and squished, and to avoid that, you've put a lot of efforts into not making any mistakes?"

"Yes."

"How has that been working out for you?" (There's our *Transition question.*)

"Not good! I am a nervous wreck."

(So there we have it! The transition questions have yielded a good result! Now onto the *Closing questions.*)

"Do you wish to continue to live this way?"

"No!"

"Is there any reason you need to continue living this way?"

"Well, I thought I have for most of my life, but now that I see where my need was coming from, I no longer need to live this way."

"So what are you going to do now?"

"I am going to stop trying to not make mistakes. I am just going to say what I need to say and let the chips fall where they may."

"Is it True?"

This is another form of a *Transition question* to ask a patient about a belief they have held to be true. It challenges them to really think about it. For example, a person states strongly, decidedly, and even confidently, albeit with misplaced confidence:

"I am always second best. In everything I do. I am placed second. My husband does it. I come second to his work. My parents placed me second best to my sister."

So the belief is clear. It's been declared. At this point, I can see where the patient is with this belief by asking the straight-shot, direct question:

"Is it true?"

If they answer, "No it's not. My mind can see it is not true, but I always keep believing it is anyway," then there is no more need for a *Transition question* at this stage, because they already see it is not true. So then it is time to further investigate. We can follow the stream by asking, *"If you can see that this is not true, what is stopping you from changing it?"* and then exploring whatever the patient declares at that point.

But what happens if the patient says, "Yes! It is true. I am always second best." Or whatever it is that they believe (negatively), is the actual truth? Then we have to ask more *Transition questions*, which challenge the positive validity of the belief, like, *"And how is that working out for you?"* If a patient is very obstinately attached to a belief, wanting to continue to hold onto it and refusing to see that it is not serving them then the practitioner has to let them go and let them continue to do so, perhaps offering homework and journaling for them to consider how it is actually serving them.

Assuming we already have the background information regarding what makes the patient believe what they believe, we don't need to ask, *"What makes you believe it is true?"* We can skip that now and go to some of the following *Transition questions*.

"How is believing you are always second best serving you?"

Or:

"What do you get out of believing you are always second best?"

Let's assume now, that the answer is, "It is not serving me." Or, "I don't get anything out of it besides heartache and frustration." So then we can move into a *Closing question* and ask, *"So do you want to keep believing it to be true?"*

They will likely say something like, "No, but..." Whatever comes after they say "but," can then be explored as part of the stream. For instance, they may say, "No, but I don't know how to change it." So then you can ask, *"What gets in the way of you knowing how to change it?"* Or, *"What have you done to try to change it?"* and then ask, *"What made that not work for you?"* Or you can ask, *"If you took a guess now, what would be a good way to change it?"*

Transition questions and *Closing questions* must also follow the basic Vis Dialogue principle of:

keeping to the context of the flow.

Another question we can ask at the point where a person seems attached to the belief is, *"What would happen if you let go of the belief you were always second best?"* This can really help to accomplish what the *Transition question* is meant to do by revealing the opposite.

"If I were to let go of the idea that I am always second best, I would feel better about myself."

"What do you think about that?"

"That would be great."

"So can we say that the idea that you are always second best limits you from feeling better about yourself?"

"Yes."

"So do you want to keep living that way?"

"No!"

"So are you going to keep living this way?"

"No!"

Then we take the patient one step further by asking, *"How is that going to look for you now in your life? How will you be applying this change?"*

Explore that with the patient and then salute them for their courage and willingness to heal themselves.

Even if a person is unable to let go of a belief because of the apparent reality of it, and the accompanying realness of the trapped emotions associated with it, it is still helpful to get them to declare that they think the belief that has controlled their lives is not true. It moves the case toward the healing direction. Most patients when asked, *"Is it true?"* about their belief will be able to recognize it is, in fact, not true. You may be the first to ever get them to ask themselves that question. It is very valuable. However, that doesn't always cause a huge impact, which shows that there are other factors that need to be addressed before the belief can be released.

Another *Transition question* that we can use following a patient's answer, "Yes, my belief is true!" is, *"Where is the evidence for it being true?"* Basically, you're getting a patient to reflect on what makes them so sure that their belief is true. Where is the evidence supporting that? From there, we can explore the source of their beliefs. If there isn't any evidence, then ask, *"So if there isn't any evidence to support the belief, then do you need to continue holding onto it?"* And if there is some "apparent" evidence to the patient, then we can challenge that evidence by asking questions to help unravel it. This will often naturally lead into *Reflecting Elsewhere* and *Transition questions* to help a patient detach from the belief as being helpful and carved in stone.

Dealing with Accompanying, Underlying Emotions with Transition Questions

Often, the other factor that is getting in the way of letting go of the belief system and needs to be released has to do with the underlying trapped/suppressed emotion that is associated with the belief. If a person has lost loved ones and are filled with buried grief, to survive, they adopted the belief that "Life is hard and I am always alone." That belief that is blocking them from living a happy life is also stopping them from feeling the grief. They are holding it like a fist in the will of their mind to avoid feeling the pain. In order to release the belief, therefore, they will have to contact and connect with the underlying grief before they feel comfortable releasing the belief "I am always alone." So here, we have to encourage people to allow themselves to feel. When I encounter a deep pocket of buried emotion, I will ask the patient what they have done or what they continue to do with the emotion, depending on the context. This is just like asking Transition questions, but for emotions. We want to help a patient see that their decision to bury or suppress the painful or difficult emotions is not in their best interest.

"What do you do with the anger?"

Many will be able to admit, "I bury it."

I will then continue to help a patient recognize if this is helping them or not.

"What happens to the anger when you bury it?"

"It just stays there."

"What is it doing while it is just staying there?"

Some will recognize the issue with the suppressed emotion right away at this point and will declare, "It's festering." Or, "It's making me sick."

Such a response makes it clear that the suppression of emotion is not serving them. If it is not clear, ask some more *Transition questions* for emotions.

"What impact does not expressing your feelings have on you?"

Or:

"How is suppressing your anger working out for you?"

"Is that something that is serving you?"

Once you've gotten them to recognize it is not serving them, it is not good; then ask the *Closing questions* in relation to the choice to suppress or bury the emotion.

"Do you want to keep burying the anger?"

"No."

"So what can you do about it then?"

Dialogue with the patient at this point about how to deal with the emotion. If it's anger, then share with them some good exercises to express their anger.

#1 – Allowing themselves to feel the anger without judgment.

ACCEPTANCE is key.

If it is possible, a healthy dialogue with the person or people that have generated the anger.

Writing them a letter and sharing it with them or burning it.

Screaming into a pillow.

Hitting a heavy bag.

Etc.

If it is sadness:

#2 – Allowing themselves to feel the sadness without judgment. ACCEPTANCE is key.

Giving themselves permission to cry. Ask them if they can do this? If not, explore what stops them. If it is beliefs adopted from their family like "Crying is a sign of weakness" or "Crying gets you nowhere", then address this as a belief system and apply *Transition* and *Closing questions* about that very belief system.

At this juncture in a case, a simple discussion and some gentle encouragement and advice can be handy where it deals with sharing something about the health benefits of allowing oneself to feel one's emotions. Asking questions to have the patients get their own answers is always preferable to giving advice, but in such a place, encouragement can work nicely, as a patient may never have heard it is ok to cry, or be angry, and they have no precedent to know it is ok without the encouragement and support from you, the practitioner. They also may not have recognized the fact that by suppressing their feelings, it causes problems for their health. Use metaphors and analogies to explain how suppressing feelings can cause problems. Something I may say, *"Think of your emotions as rivers that flow around in your body. What happens when you put a dam on a river?"* You can let them answer. I then also say, *"It all builds up on one side, and causes a dryness on the other side. Two extremes that are very unbalanced. So we want to remove the dam that is suppressing our emotions. Does that make sense to you?"*

"What will you do now?"

"How is that going to look?"

"How are you going to live from now on?"

After a person has decided to let go of a belief, it is time to explore the next steps into the future that they will take. We can use these three questions to do so, such as, *"So what is that going to look like for you?"*

Some answers can be akin to "I am no longer going to allow my brother to treat me the way he does."

"What will you do?"

"I am going to have a talk with him and set some very clear boundaries that he does not have the right to treat me so disrespectfully."

"Can you do it?"

This is a *Closing question* to have a person reflect on whether they can make the change and let go of the old belief system. For example, we have gotten to the core belief, and past the *Transition questions*. The patient does not want to continue living believing that they are good for nothing. They have just said, "No. I do not want to continue believing I am good for nothing."

So the next *Closing question* we can ask here is, *"So can you let go of believing that you are good for nothing?"* If they say, "No. I cannot let it go." Then ask, *"What is stopping you?"* and explore that direction. If they say, "Yes! I can let it go now."

Then ask **"Will *you* do it?"**

Hopefully, they say yes. In fact, at this point, it would be silly to say, "Yes, I can let it go." To then state, "Yes, I can, but I am not going to." So the *"Will you do it?"* *Closing question* is just a formality to get the patient to deepen a commitment to change. They should say, "Yes!"

When they get to the bottom line and say yes, I am going to change, I always say things like "Good. Excellent. Good for you! That's so brave. You're so good at this." Depending on the nature of the patient and what sort of "pat on the back" may serve them best as encouragement to support them in their newfound choices.

Here I would again congratulate, support, and possibly ask, *"How does that feel for you?"*

The "I AM" of the soul and the Heart's Desire

Once a person's belief is gone, how do they decide what to be? How to be? The answer to this is quite interesting. In the beginning of the book, I shared how the I AM statement emerges from the soul. It is an expression of each of our true natures. But how do we recognize and understand our unique I AM statements? How do we know who we really are? The answer itself emerges from the soul, from the I AM statement. Once the false belief system is released, there should be an effortless, natural alignment that happens with the person's I AM. The false belief was simply occluding, dampening, and getting in the way of the person knowing their true self. When that false opposition is removed, Nature should be restored. And so at the point in the dialogue when we ask, *"What will you do now?"* Or, *"How do you want to be from here on out?"* a person normally spontaneously and rather effortlessly has a sense of what they'd like to do. And here is where the heart's desire comes into the picture. In my awareness, the way we hear our I AM statement is through the desire of the heart. This is rather simple, yet the explanation is quite profound.

Carl Jung stated:

Man can try to name love, showering upon it all the names at his command, and he will still involve himself in endless self-deceptions. If he possesses a grain of wisdom, he will lay down his arms and name the unknown by the more unknown: by the name of God.[19]

Here we recall that the soul is One with God, the Creator. And God is Love. So, that means that our true Nature is also Love.

And here is a very simple, yet most beautiful awareness. How do we know our soul? How do we know our I AM? We know our I AM and our soul by how we *love* to be, and by what we *love* to do. Because our very essence is Love, our Nature speaks to us and guides us through that very essence.

In my book, *Book 1 of The Last Four Books of Moses*, on Kabbalah, I wrote a phrase that portrays this relationship between soul and how we choose to align with its calling, as follows:

I choose to be because I love to be.
So I allow myself to be, because I know I AM.[20]

That which we love to be, is that which we are, otherwise, why would we love to be it?

I've often been asked by students and patients, "How do I know my life's purpose?" Sometimes people have gone so long disconnected from themselves that they even ask, "How do I know who I am?"

The answer is – You know who you are by what you *love to be*. That's it. Plain and simple. This "love to be" is felt as the desire of the heart. This desire is a true desire. The first of the *Two Paths*. The path of Truth. The path of the heart. It is healthy. Inspiring. soulful. It connects the soul on its true path. This is not the *second path*. It is not the desire of the ego to run from fear. It is a true and natural desire. Sometimes, yes, the desire has been deeply buried. But it is always there. No matter how far a person has strayed from the path of the heart, they can always find it again and reclaim it.

So at this point in the dialogue, when all that is left is to encourage a patient to choose how they are going to be from here on in, (which is truly more of an alignment and "an allowing" than a choice), knowing that their soul has the answer is very edifying. If a patient is so unclear and uncertain how they intend on being, you can ask, *"How would you most love to be now?"* that is a very wise question. If they still have no idea and are unable to make that connection with their heart's desire, ask them, *"Can you remember how you used to love to be, when you were younger?"* This can help a patient remember how they used to be spontaneously, before they allowed the false beliefs to block out their I AM.

I will also ask, *"Can you remember your dreams?"* These are not the dreams one has during sleep, but the hopes and dreams one has had (11th house in astrology). This is a clue toward helping the patient remember who they really are.

We are what we love to be.

Acceptance and Forgiveness

New question: *"Can you accept that?"*

Sometimes, the path to freedom for a patient may be blocked by great bitterness and hatred from having suffered wrong at the hands of another, or others, or from a very difficult situation. Before any letting go and healing can occur, the person must *first accept* and *then forgive* the person that hurt them.

This question is directive in nature. It is asking a person, when they are speaking of something very difficult, if they can accept it. It comes from the understanding that acceptance is the first step to healing. Without acceptance, a person continues to fight against what they judge. This leaves them always and perpetually in relationship to what they are judging. When they accept something they don't like, then they can let go.

Sometimes, I need to explain the difference between accepting something as in "not judging it" from saying, "I am ok with it and I am ok if it never goes away." That is not acceptance. That is giving away one's heart's desire to be healthy and happy. True acceptance involves, in the simplest sense, recognizing the existence of something as being there, without judging it, fighting it, and trying to destroy it. In others words, I am simply accepting the fact that this is there. I cannot deny it any longer. Acceptance, therefore, is no more than *stopping oneself from denying something*, but the effects are far reaching and worth the endeavor.

Once acceptance is in place, forgiveness can follow. I find it is difficult for someone to forgive another that has hurt them when they first have not accepted what that person has done. "I cannot believe my mother did that to me. I will never forgive her." Forgiveness is sometimes very hard to get at to begin with. Without acceptance, it is almost impossible. The "I cannot believe" is a sign that acceptance has not yet entered into the situation.

"Can you accept that your mother did do what she did?"

If a person says, "No, I cannot accept that." Then you can dialogue about that specific answer. *"What makes you not be able to accept what your mother did to you?"*

Or you may simply need to say, *"Without acceptance, it is very difficult to let go of unhealthy emotions that are stuck from such difficult situations."*

In simple terms, healing involves 1) Awareness/recognition. 2) Acceptance. 3) Change. Without awareness, there can be no acceptance. Without acceptance, there can be no change.

Forgiveness, on the other hand, is like the purple heart of woundedness. It's a sign that the person was indeed wounded, but that they are out of the war. When a person is able to release the ill effects that others have done to them through forgiveness, they have evolved beyond the negativity of the situation. In that way, they are healed and do not need to grind it out with the person by remaining in a negative situation or in the remnants and memories of the negative situation. They have graduated and can move on.

The 'Name it and Cross it off' Technique

Earlier, I shared a form of a question as follows: *"So of all the things you just mentioned... which of those do you feel carries the most weight/impact?"*

This was in response to someone expressing several feelings or issues at the same time. "When someone breaks up with me, I feel alone, scared, angry and like a failure." So we will ask them which has the most weight so that we can go deepest down the *Rabbit Hole* and through the most weighted negativity they are experiencing. The *Name it and Cross it off technique* is similar, but arises when someone lists a number of reasons why they cannot let go of a thought or a behavior pattern.

For example, in one case, I was dialoguing with a woman who was thinking of leaving her husband. We arrived at the point in the dialogue where she stated, "I do feel I would like to move on."

"So what is stopping you from moving on?"

"Well, what would my neighbors think? What will my parents think? Where will I find the money to survive? How will I manage being all alone?"

Like in the *"What carries the most weight?"* topic, one could ask *"Which of these concerns carries the most weight?"* However, that is not really helpful at this point because they have stated four reasons that are stopping them. Each must be explored. So what I do is give them feedback and state the following, even taking a piece of paper to jot down the four (or however many) points they state:

"So you said, "What would my neighbors think? What will my parents think? Where will I find the money to survive? How will I manage being all alone?" Let's jot these down here (on the piece of paper) and explore them one at a time." Then I will begin with the first one on the list and ask:

"So what is the worst thing that your neighbors could think?"

And then explore from then on what is underlying that concern and each subsequent concern.

Another thing we can do, at the point of receiving the four or however many concerns that are stopping a person from living what they want, is to ask them which has the most weight.

"Which of these concerns has the most weight for you? Let's explore that one first." And then when that is resolved, cross it off the list and ask which one has the next most weight and explore that.

It can take a while to explore and cross off four points on a list. Some may easily be dismissed. Some may open up large issues that a person didn't even realize they were going to be discussing in relation to ending a marriage, or whatever their issue was. One of the points can open up such a large journey into the Rabbit Hole that it can take an entire session.

So when exploring each of the points, one could ask something as follows, *"So what is the worst thing that your neighbors could think?"*

"Well, they could think I wasn't a very good Christian."

"And what if they didn't think you were a good Christian?"

"Well, tough on them! I know I am ok, and besides, they're not the perfect Christians either. So let them think what they want."

So then I will say, *"So do you feel comfortable with this issue now?"*

"Yes. I guess it's not such a big deal after all."

So then I will cross it off the list, which leaves three more issues.

"Ok. So let's move on to the next issue on the list. What would your parents think? What is the worst thing you can imagine them thinking?"

"They'll think that I am letting them down."

This is something that can use some exploration.

"What makes you think that?"

"My parents always used to feel disappointed when I wouldn't succeed at something."

"Is that what you think would happen now?"

A possible simple answer: "Well, now that I think of it, they'll want me to be happy. So probably not."

"So is this still an issue, i.e. what your parents would think?"

Answer: "No. It's not really an issue."

So we can cross off that issue from the list, which leaves us with two more.

More complicated answer: "Yes, I feel I'd be letting them down if I ended my marriage."

From here, we'll have to pull out some of the big questions we've already learned to get to the bottom of this point.

"And what if you let them down? What would come up for you if you felt you did?"

(Here's another example of two questions asked at the same time.)

So here is the bottom line of this exercise. Ask someone what is stopping them from changing their belief? They state a list. Write down the list. Explore each issue, one at a time. When an issue is resolved, when it has been "seen through" and is no longer a problem, then cross it off the list. When all the issues have been resolved, bring it back to the original question.

"So all of these issues you brought up were in response to the question, "What is stopping you from walking away?" And we have explored each one together and you have felt comfortable that these are non-issues now. So is there anything stopping you now from walking away?"

Here a patient should say, "No." Say *"Excellent!"* and then ask:

"So what are you going to do now?"

Each case will yield different results at each of these stages. For my patient that actually listed those four things, after we got to the end of the list, she realized there was nothing stopping her from walking away. What that brought up for her was the realization that she did not really want to walk away. Once the fears that seemed to be stopping her from walking away were cleared, and she felt free to walk away, she actually recognized the fact that she didn't want to leave after all. Maybe that was still just fear of walking away and *the Second path* seeming more appealing than the *First*. Whatever the case, I don't normally give my opinion about whether or not someone should walk away from their partner, whether it be a girlfriend, boyfriend, or a spouse. People can get into quite a tizzy in regards to staying in or leaving a relationship. They feel confused, pulled in many directions at once. Many of their core issues are brought up. They will often ask, "What do you think?" It's tempting to give one's opinion. I will say, *"How should I know what is right for you? What do you feel? What is stopping you from knowing what is right for you?"* I did once have a case where a woman was desperate to know what to do. She asked me, repeatedly, despite my several attempts to say that I don't like to give advice, what she should do. I finally said, *"In this situation, I would choose to be true to myself."* It sort of hinted at which path to walk, because she had said a few times that she felt it was being true to herself to walk away. I didn't say, *"I would walk away."* I said, *"I would choose to be true to myself"* which could be applied in any situation. Even though people may be desperate for the answers, they may seem content if you give them the answers right away. But if you can refrain from giving them the answers and instead guide them to finding the right answer for themselves they will be much happier about it and will really appreciate your help in the matter. It's also quite alright to leave them with some unanswered questions.

As another example of *the Name It and Cross it off Technique*, we get down to the bottom line with a patient who believes they can only trust and rely on themselves. Nobody else. This is mostly in relation to having a romantic partnership. There is also a history of being stalked, and of having been with very unsafe people that were not trustworthy (real situation). After some of the *Transition questions* like, *"How is that working out for you?"* and,

"What would your life be like if you didn't believe you were the only one you could trust and rely on?" we get down to the *Closing question: "Do you want to keep living this way?"*

And she says, "No."

"So are you going to keep living this way?"

"I'm not sure. I don't know."

"What's stopping you from changing this about yourself?"

"How will I know if someone is good or bad for me? How will I ever let someone know where my house is? What if they try to rape me or take advantage of me?"

So obviously, even after having gotten to the bottom line belief, there are quite a few issues still lingering. The emotional trauma is still sticking to the patient, as well as other traumas that have emotionally upheld the belief that she cannot trust anyone but herself. So these are very legitimate concerns that she has before she feels comfortable letting go of her belief systems. Each point brought up must be examined closely, so that the fears can be brought to the surface and scrutinized. This helps call up the emotion and if done gently, and patiently, can help a person let go of the past and be ready to choose a new and healthier path for themselves.

We would get out the list and say, *"Ok, here are the things that seem to be getting in the way of you deciding to change the way you've been deciding to do things. Let's explore the first thing on the list first. How do you normally know if someone is good or bad?"*

"Well, that's just it. I have trusted my intuition but it's been wrong about people."

(This is almost a blank-stare, open-mouthed answer. This often is the result of a "real situation." The practitioner is thinking "Yeah, that's what I'd think too." Or "I can really understand where they're coming from." Nevertheless, there is an opening somewhere to go deeper. It may require a gutsy question, to challenge the seemingly obviousness of their reply.

In any case, her last answer needs to be explored further.)

"Tell me more about that." (Always a good question when we're still in the "blank stare" phase.)

"There've been times when I've thought someone was good, but they ended up being a bad person."

*"You **thought** they were good? Or it was your intuition telling you they were good?"*

(This is directive, yet necessary to discern the difference, since she just stated that her intuition has been wrong and here she stated she thought. So I picked up on that discrepancy, found it strange, and so I asked her about that.)

"I thought they were good."

"What made you think they were good?"

"Now that I think back, I can see I wanted to think they were good."

"What made you do that?"

"They flattered me and told me how beautiful I am. I am a sucker for that and I throw all logic, and reasoning, and even my intuition away."

"So can we say that you've allowed yourself to not see or discern whether a person was bad for you because they flattered you?"

"Yup. That pretty much is true."

"Were there any signs or instincts about the last person that this happened with?"

"Yes, there were. There was something about him I really didn't like. But I chose to ignore that when he began flattering me."

"Are you going to keep doing that in the future?"

"No. I won't do that anymore."

"So do you feel comfortable with the issue now of, How will I know if someone is good or bad for me?"

Answer: "Yes."

"Can we cross it off the list?"

Answer: "Yes."

So we can cross it off and move on to the next item on the list. Let's assume we were able to explore and cross each item off the list. Then we'll bring it back to the original *Closing question*: "*So is there anything else that is stopping you from letting go of the idea that you're the only one you can trust and rely on?*"

"No! There isn't."

"*Great! So what are you going to do now?*" Or, "*So are you going to keep living this way?*"

"I am going to meet someone and discern whether or not they are a good person for me. I will not let myself fall for flattery if I sense something is not good about them for me. And, I will allow myself to trust them."

This is great! It is a clear and concise answer and a declaration of change. At this point, it is time for a little celebration.

"*Good for you! That is so excellent. That's fantastic! What an amazing declaration.*"

Now, give it room to breathe and grow into a more "firm/formed" reality. You can just chat about it at this point, casually, allowing for the new-found truth to settle into place even further. Encourage them to see the far-reaching implications for their life.

Vis Dialogue Summary until Now

So for now, in our understanding of the Holistic Counseling Vis Dialogue, we have: **Ask non-directive questions, go with the flow by asking the next open-ended question that naturally presents itself from the last thing the person said, keep to the context of the flow, use directive questions only at key points, and occasionally give feedback, all the while remembering the important principle of going into and through the negative. If a** *blank-stare, open-mouthed wall* **is encountered, keep on going. Ask** *Reflecting Elsewhere* **questions to help a person see their belief is not carved in stone. Once the underlying/core belief is** exposed, ask *Transition questions* to help a patient detach from their belief before asking *Closing questions*. Once a person decides they will let go of their belief, ask them how they plan on being from then on.

Stated even more simply.

Expose the belief (the main Holistic Counseling Vis Dialogue questions).

Recognize the belief is not carved in stone (*Reflecting Elsewhere* questions).

Declare the belief as negative and no longer serving (*Transition questions*).

Help the person to change their mind & unchoose their belief (*Closing questions*).

Summary of the Questions that were shared in Chapter 29, 30, 31

Chapter 29: "What's the opposite of that? What would the opposite feel like?"

Reflecting Elsewhere question Part 2: "What is common between these situations?"

Reflecting on Past, which is related to, "Is it true?" for eg: "Now that you're thinking about it, do you think that you were stupid those times when you said something he didn't like or agree with?"

"How is that working out for you?" (Transition question.)

"How did you respond to that? What was your response to that? How did you react to that sort of situation?"

"What do you do with that? What comes after that?"

"So you feel "x", for example, angry or sad or nervous, what do you do when you feel that? What is the next thing that you do when you're feeling angry/sad/nervous?"

"Can you see where you have misinterpreted something there? What would you have done differently?"

"What do you think/feel motivated that person to be the way

they were with you?"

Questions with an Observation: – *"I noticed that you're (for e.g) crossing your arms, touching your face, closing your eyes tightly, clenching your jaw, not breathing, playing with your clothes, moving your feet back and forth? What's going on there for you?"* or, *"What is making you do that?"*

When people express things vaguely: *The Pot Metaphor*

"Imagine the "terrible" or the "bad" feeling is a pot, now throw it on the ground and let it all break open. What do you see inside of the pot? What is in there inside the bad and the terrible?"

"What if you didn't believe that? What would your life be like if you didn't believe that?"

Boiling down a Belief – Helping a Patient to Isolate a Belief or a Behavior Pattern

Isolating Conditional I AM Statements

"So can we say, "I have a good job, therefore I Am?""

"So can we say, "I have children, therefore I Am?""

Take a Guess Technique

Chapter 30: Investigating a Physical Condition:

LOCATION – SENSATION – MODALITIES (is a general set of questions to ask).

"Where is the issue located? Does it radiate anywhere else?"

CAUSE/ONSET –

"What brings it on (exciting cause), what triggers it?"

"What and when makes it get better or worse?"

Accompanying Symptoms

"Are there any symptoms that come along with the condition?" (These can also be mental-emotional symptoms.)

"How long have you had them?"

"How is it affected by: Light, which foods, eating, exercise, sex, touch, pressure, weather, alone or in a group, sound, stress (what kind of stress)?"

"How does the illness feel?" Literally, how does it feel?

Important for Going Deeper and Establishing a Connection with the Root Cause:

"How do you feel about it? Or how does your condition make you feel?"

Related to when it began:

"When did it begin? What was happening at the time? Was there anything that happened out of the ordinary during your life right around or just before that time that you got sick?"

"How do you feel about the illness?" It's like asking, *"How do you feel about the fact that you have the illness?"* Or, *"How do you feel since you have the illness?"*

When the feeling of the illness leads to something that sounds like it points to the life:

"Is there anywhere else in your life that makes you feel that way?"

And:

"What did you feel right before or during the injury?"

Dealing with Accompanying, Underlying Emotions with Transition Questions

"What do you do with the anger?"

"What happens to the anger when you bury it?"

"What is it doing while it is just staying there?"

"Do you want to keep burying the anger?"

"So what can you do about it then?"

"Can you Accept That?"

The 'Name it and Cross it off' Technique

Chapter 31) Closing Questions and Closing Situations

Transition (into Closing) questions

"How's that working out for you?"

"What are you getting out of believing that?"

"How does it serve you?"

"Is it True?"

Closing questions:

"Do you want to keep living that way?"
"Is this how you want to be?"
"Is this who you really are?"
"What's stopping you from letting that go?"
"What's stopping you from changing that idea or pattern?"
"Are you ready to let that go?"
"Are you going to let that go?"
"How are you going to live from now on?"

Chapter 32

What to Do When the Case is not Advancing or is Stuck

A case can grind to a halt at a certain point or can never even get off the ground to begin with. When I say it never even gets off the ground, it means the questions don't lead anywhere. Nothing opens up. It's like continuously hitting a wall. Also, I like to use the metaphor of questions going down *the Rabbit Hole*. This is *vertical* movement down deeper into the person's psyche via the questions. When a person just tells stories and then more stories of an external nature, they are speaking and spreading out *horizontally*. This does not help move deeper into a person. When this occurs, either during a given dialogue, or in the long run between follows-ups, there are certain things that a practitioner can do to help the case move forward. One thing I will do is actually explain this to the patient. I'll say, *"You're filling me in about a lot of information in your life. You're telling me the story. It's good for me to get a general sense of the context of the story surrounding your struggles and issues. The telling of the story provides me with information on what I call 'the horizontal plane.' However, what I know to be most helpful for people is to go deeper, by answering questions that enable us to connect to how you're really feeling and what you're struggling with in your subconscious. That is what I call going deeper on the 'vertical plane.' So let's limit how much horizontal information you provide so that we can get you to go deeper, vertically. Ok?"*

In truth, not much context at all is needed to help set a person free. You can jump right into how a person is feeling and what they believe about the situation. But the patient feels they need to share that at least enough so that the situation is understood.

That's fine. I let patients do that and it does help to be more involved so that it is not too vague for me. But when they begin telling me too many details of the 'horizontal' kind, that's when I intervene and give them the horizontal vs vertical spiel.

Now, let's look at what to do when a case is not advancing during an actual dialogue, then we will look at when the patient is not improving or recovering in the long run despite the fact that the Vis Dialogue has been going well during the appointments.

In some cases, a patient gives very little information. They don't seem to want to answer any questions, or their answers are, "Fine." "No problem." "I don't know." "That doesn't bother me." "Nothing's wrong." "It's all good" and they give you no additional information, ideas, feelings, or anything that you can work with. Such a case may fall under "The Limitations of Holistic Counseling" in that they are simply not a very good candidate for Holistic Counseling. However, I have had some cases seem very stuck and like an immovable object, and with enough questions, directed creatively and from different "angles," the patient did open up and the case did progress. So I do not recommend giving up at the first sign of immovability, but rather endeavoring to get past the present obstacles that restrict a patient from making progress. Some people are just not used to the process and need some time to grasp what you're really asking. Others are unsure about the whole process and need to warm up. Given time, they will open up.

If after asking many questions that are answered something akin to, "I am fine." "Nah, no problem there." "That doesn't bother me," you may need to ask a reminder question, *"What did you come here for?"* Hearing them say what condition or illness made them choose to come for the visit and having them state or restate a commitment to get healthy can be important in some cases. Having them repeat the purpose of the visit is important, because sometimes the illness desires to survive and that can overpower a patient's conscious intention to heal themselves. It's almost as if they want to get better, so they book an appointment, but then, once they sit down and you begin dialoguing with them, they are so very in the moment, that they have already forgotten that they want to heal and rather, their desire to avoid their problems takes charge and dominates their psyche. So asking them, *"May I ask you again what it is that brought you here?"* may help get through to the person's cooperative healing mode, rather than their denial and avoidance mode.

Sometimes, I will ask a patient straight out, *"Do you know what your problem is?"*

Be aware that the intention behind it is important; it is not to be brought across at all as blaming and try not to sound like Robert De Niro's character in the movie *The Godfather*. But just cutting to the chase can, at times, reveal important jewels.

If they are really stuck, you may need to ask the patient:

"Do you really wish to heal?"

"Are you sure you wish to heal?"

Ask with sincerity and compassion, and also directness.

Imagine that they are sent by a loved one and do not really want to be there and all the lack of answers that you're experiencing is due to that fact. The complete lack of helpful answers is a red flag that can mean that the patient does not want to a) be there at all or b) heal.

If it is that they do not want to be there, it is important that the practitioner gives them the freedom to leave. I have seen that when freedom is offered, the person now has the option to remain, if they want, *of their own accord*. That is key and can make the entire difference.

If the answer is that they don't want to heal then think of looking for or searching out for a reason that they have invested in being sick. Sometimes this is a process that is not initiated by the patient. Rather, the practitioner may have gotten some indication or even a possible intuitive feeling that the patient does not want to heal.

Think of the self-supportive syndromes. For example, many people that feel very angry do not want to let go of the anger because it is giving them something. It could be that it makes them feel powerful when they really feel disempowered or powerless inside. Or the very fact that they feel angry means that they are angry about something and so will not like to let go of that anger until what they are angry about resolves. Sometimes people want to hold onto the cause of their problem for a specific reason. For example, someone is holding onto grief. This has led to their illness, but they do not want to let go of the grief because they do not want to say goodbye to the person they have lost. So, letting go of the grief, which would lead to healing, also means that they must let go of their loved one. And so since healing means letting go of their loved one, they don't want to heal. This needs to be brought out in the dialogue and discussed. Just bringing the conundrum to the attention of a patient can be enough to get the case to move forward again.

Sometimes people have an attitude that states, "I've been doing it this way for so long, surely, someday, it will pay off, or I will succeed." The idea there is that they cannot let go of how they are choosing to live because they've been going at it for so long that letting go and surrendering means that all that time was for naught. What a waste! What a devastating loss of time, energy, and effort. This is a very painful reason that people do not want to progress and the awareness must be brought about gently, and firmly, and with a lot of compassion.

A practitioner may need to look for the "candy" of why they are holding on to their illness.

For example, some people are still "Looking for mommy or daddy's approval." This dynamic can be crippling for a person because the very thing that is harming them is what they do not want to let go of. Some controlling parents discover that by not approving of a child's behavior, by constantly disapproving and finding fault in their child's behavior, they can always have that child running around trying to please them. This makes the parent feel respected and powerful (as a compensation for how they really feel about themselves). It is a very unhealthy, narcissistic form of parenting that leads their children to have serious problems later on in life. Now, from time to time, the parent will acknowledge the child has done well, but it is only if the child has done it in such a fashion that the parent deems worthy. Therefore, the only time the child sees the parent offering anything that resembles love, is when they have pleased their parents by doing just what their parents wanted. This behavior is often perpetuated well into life. And there you have a patient, who is poised for change, not wanting to change, because to let go of the unhealthy behavior of doing what others want (because of their parents' narcissistic behavior) means to let go of the one thing that they think brings them love. This must be revealed through the Vis Dialogue. If it is not quite getting through, the practitioner may need to illustrate and explain the situation in plain terms so that the patient can understand.

Another reason that someone wants to remain sick is that people feel sorry for them because they are sick. Some people never feel heard, or understood, or cared for, except when they are sick. I have several patients whose parents didn't show any sign of affection or love unless they were sick. Who can blame them for growing up and becoming attached to being sick to gain love and attention?

In the case of a woman in her seventies who was attached to being sick because it was the only time her mother showed her any signs of compassion and care, she was also attached to feeling like she didn't matter, and that nobody cared about her. When we explored deeper, it became clear that she was actually attached to the belief that she was a victim. Being a victim, although it sounds entirely negative, actually had some form of candy attached to it for her. It was very interesting to discover this and reminded me again of just how very strong the imagination of a child is. That child becomes the inner child of an adult and continues to hold onto ideas that are often completely unrealistic and ungrounded, but very imaginative and creative.

So this patient was attached to being a victim because she felt it was her identity. Her older brother was the "older one." Her other siblings got labeled as the smart one, the musical one, and the good athlete. This woman felt like nobody cared about her and almost as if she didn't exist. However, being a victim gave her some sort of identity that she then became attached to. Exposing this through the dialogue and subsequently helping her release it, enabled her to move past a majority of the reason behind her being sick.

In some cases patients don't want to have to return to work. They hate their job but don't know how to get out of it, and so it is only through debilitating symptoms that they gain the reason to get out of their jobs.

In all these different cases where there is candy or something preventing the patient from making progress in their healing, the practitioner should first help reveal the fact through the Vis Dialogue, and if that doesn't arise naturally, give some feedback to make it clear that the belief is actually getting in the way of accomplishing their ultimate goals (getting better), and then by posing the *Transition* and *Closing questions* to get them to release that obstacle in their path to health.

At times during the interview, there is not always some profound underlying blockage and resistance or candy that a patient is holding onto, but simply, *the Rabbit Hole* that was being explored turns up to be a dead end that led nowhere or you hit a wall and there's no getting around it no matter how many creative and specialized questions you use. At such a point, I recommend that you change the topic completely towards a) what they may have mentioned previously that may have peaked your curiosity; b) a topic you intuitively feel is important c) a topic that they visited (e.g. work, home, siblings, children, spouse, etc.) that you sensed had some emotional charge attached to it. As a practitioner develops their listening skills and they are relaxed, they can pick up subtle signs from the patient that may escape someone with less experience or who is preoccupied with doing the technique rather than observing. At times, I sense a change in the patient's voice when they are discussing a certain area in their life which makes it clear that there is something difficult or painful there for them. For example, "I go to work, I come home, I see the kids, I prepare dinner *for my husband*, then I go see my friends, I do the laundry, etc., etc." When this particular person said, "for my husband" the jaw clenched slightly, and the voice changed, as if the person was holding back a little bird that wanted to escape from their throat. But then the person continues talking and the moment to ask about that is gone, without needing to interrupt the flow. I will make a little note next to that part of the text to revisit it later, if we hit a dead end and need something else to explore.

During a dialogue, I always make a mental note of things I want to go back to, to investigate. It helps me to actually mark a note next to the place. I use the letters *xix* in my word document because there is no word that has *xix* in it, so a quick search in Microsoft Word for *xix* will bring up the special note and it all takes about two seconds and is not disruptive to the flow of the Dialogue. But really, any letters that do not exist could be used as a bookmark, such as zzz or ttt.

Movies as a Means of Connection

Sometimes, people don't like the awkwardness of being asked personal questions about themselves. Who knows? Maybe they were raised in a family where they learned that it wasn't polite to ask personal questions. Or they may simply feel uncomfortable being on the spot and so they are freezing up and not answering your questions. Here, I'll use a simple trick to take a less direct approach, which can ease the pressure a little bit. I'll ask about their favorite movie and then ask what was so special to them about that movie? Then question them about it and move into a dialogue seamlessly. This can help to assuage the shyness they may have at meeting a stranger. Talking about a movie is much less threatening to them than speaking directly about their own personal problems. It's a means to create a bridge. For example, *"What's your favorite movie?"*

"Beaches."

"What is it about Beaches that makes it your favorite movie?"

"It helps me to cry."

"Do you have a difficulty crying otherwise?"

"Yes."

"When did that start for you?"

So we see it can be a good opportunity to go from awkward, no-info responses, to getting the person to open up a little about themself. As another example:

"What's your favorite movie?"

"Fight Club."

"What did you like about Fight Club?"

"I loved how the men were being so masculine, such real men."

"What would be the opposite of that – of men being masculine and real men?"

"It would be where a man is not allowed to be strong."

"What would make a man not allowed to be strong?"

"If there was always someone putting him down whenever he tried to be assertive, strong."

"Is that true for you?"

"Yes."

Aha! So we have "gotten in there" and moved from a movie to actual life. Often, a person's favorite movie will actually provide this bridge or a gateway into their inner feelings.

Dreams into Waking Life Technique

Similar to asking about movies is asking about recurrent dreams
they may have had. This is even more powerful than the movies
because the dreams are direct expressions of the subconscious
mind. The most important dreams are those that occur more than
once, and the ones that have themes repeated. So for instance,
some dreams are more or less identical. They are recurrent
dreams. These are the best to explore for this purpose. Even if the
case is not stuck, I like to ask about recurrent dreams as we gain
a beeline to the patient's subconscious. A recurrent theme in the
dream would have dreams sharing a theme but not necessarily
looking all the same. For instance, a person may dream one night
of being on a tall building and then falling off, and in another
dream, they could be in a totally different situation, but will still
fall off of some high object, or fall down into some deep pit.
Another example is that the patient may dream of being trapped
without any means of escape, despite the surrounding circumstances of the dreams looking quite different. So the theme of
falling or being trapped with no escape is shared and becomes
the important recurrence that is like the thread in Holistic
Counseling. This is what should be focused on and explored in
the dream.

I may ask about some of the details of the dream to get a
better sense of the dream. Then I ask them how they felt in the
dream. I ask the Vis Dialogue questions concerning feelings as if
it is in a regular dialogue. For example they say:

"I feel trapped in the dream."

"What is the trapped feeling like for you in the dream?"

"It's very uncomfortable, like there is no way out."

"Tell me about what it is like to have no way out."

"It's like very dark and like everything is closing in on me."

"How do you feel when everything is closing in on you?"

"I feel panicky. Like I stop thinking rationally and instead just
don't do anything to find a way out."

"Tell me about how you stop thinking rationally?"

"It's like when I choose to panic, then I get so scared, I 'curl up within myself' and stop feeling like I can find a way out. It's like I give up."

After doing such an exploration for a given time, when the answers begin to sound like the person is talking about something in their waking life, I will then ask the question:

"Is there anywhere in your waking life that makes you feel this way?"

Just like the *Exploring-Elsewhere questions* to establish a connection between a physical condition and a mind-body connection to their life, while exploring dreams, it becomes clear that the subconscious mind and the associated emotions in the dream are a reflection of waking life. When I ask them if there is anything that makes them feel that way in their life, if they say yes, then we continue to follow that stream and establish what struggle or trouble the dream is representing in their waking life.

The *dream into waking life* technique is one of my favorite techniques in Holistic Counseling. I'll use this a lot even when the case is not stuck, to just gather even deeper information and sometimes, to find a deep vein in the Rabbit Hole that was not arrived at by following the stream. It is also extremely helpful for finding homeopathic remedies that are deep expressions of the Vital Force mistunement. One could get into the habit of always asking about recurrent dreams or repeated themes in dreams.

Another area that can also be explored when the time is right is the fear of death. It is always good to explore. What is the fear of death really about for someone? It gives a great insight into the nature of a person's issue and fear.

Prayer & Divine Assistance

Ask for Divine assistance. It really works. I sometimes pray openly with patients, especially if it is in their spiritual practices and beliefs to do so. I try to make it a practice to pray before every appointment, and when I forget, or where I hit great difficulty, I will speak a quiet prayer right at the time of difficulty. And more often than not, help is on the way. The case will open up. The questions go smoother. Answers are more forthcoming. I have also noticed that when I pray for Divine assistance before or during an appointment, I will more easily find good remedies for my patients.

When there is a "stuck" element that will not go away: The Hold it For Longer Technique

When you get to a stuck element in the case, perhaps an emotion, or a difficult idea or feeling, you can encourage them to "Do it more. To hold it longer." Do the illness more. Accentuate the holding on further. Eat the whole chocolate cake. Charge into the valley of death. This is especially true of a stuck emotion that is being repressed or avoided. By allowing oneself to feel it, it can move and be released. Also, when we look at how the mind chooses to hold onto a belief system, when we dive into the will to hold onto a belief system and we *do it more*, and then keep holding it and doing it more, somehow, the will to then actually hold onto the belief system is diminished and it becomes easier to let go. Like with the child with a weight problem who wishes to eat chocolate cake, the desire is strong to eat chocolate cake. Forbidding the child to eat the chocolate cake only makes that desire stronger. (Adam and Eve did eat from the Tree of Knowledge despite God saying it is the only tree they should not eat from, didn't they?) However, by not only allowing the child to do so, but making them eat the whole chocolate cake, it can change the will from wanting to do something, to not wanting to do it at all. A friend of mine told me that when his father caught him smoking as a child, his father made him smoke an entire pack of cigarettes, non-stop, one after the other. It was so overwhelming and disgusting to my friend, that he never smoked cigarettes again.

Also, we subconsciously fight with our illness by opposing it, resisting it, and fighting with it without being aware of it. This leads to an inherent judgment within us. And I believe that anything that is judged is given a form of empowerment from the Universe to have the right to exist. So what occurs when we wilfully charge into the illness or issue and hold it for longer is that the opposition to the illness and corresponding judgment of it as bad is lifted. It then can be released. Illness has a firmer grip when we oppose it and judge it. This exercise is a form of putting acceptance into action.

Stuckness in a Case in the Long Run Perspective

When the case is not advancing or getting stuck in the long run, then the practitioner has to do a little investigation and determine what it is that is blocking the further progress of the case. Is there an obstacle to cure? Is there a deep underlying element to the case that has yet to be addressed? Are the patients seeing other practitioners that are just treating the symptoms and letting the patient off the hook of responsibility for self?

I have had several cases that would do amazingly well during the interview only to return with the same problems during a follow-up. We would go very deeply and a belief system would be revealed and released. The patient would leave the appointment feeling better, happier, more hopeful, and then, during the first ten seconds of our follow-up, it would be clear to me that they were back where they started. Negative. Hopeless. Stuck. One thing that these patients had in common was that they saw a lot of other practitioners and/or they did a lot of research to find solutions in the form of pills, supplements, and nutritional changes. It's like, in my presence, they would follow the path of Holism, but once out of my office, they would revert to looking for an "outside" solution. I would listen to them describe these special supplements or cutting edge pills they had found on the internet or heard about that are supposed to be great for their condition, or that their doctor or other alternative healthcare practitioner had given them. After listening to this, I would begin to ask questions about their symptoms and we would arrive at the same place as last time. They would see the mind-body connection, choose to not do the false belief and negative behavior anymore, and then see the immediate change in their entire system. After a while, I realized some people are so deeply ingrained with the idea that they either cannot do the healing themselves because they feel incapable, or they simply do not want to. So when they are presented with an easy fix, the deeply insightful, empowering awareness they've discovered during our appointments goes out the window. It's like the moth of their inner self is attracted to the bright fancy lights of the allopathic world of the quick fix. With the promising offer of something that will take away their problem, without them having to do anything about it, they are happy to give away their power. Something in them wants to be subject to, rather than empowered by. There's not much the practitioner can do about it, because the changes have to come from the patient. And then I also discovered that many of these patients, having a lack of belief in themselves, do not feel that they can do anything *on their own*. The very thought of healing the self thus becomes nullified in the world because they have a baseline idea that they are incapable. All the pills, protocols, and supplements thus become their little helpers, the supports that they need because they feel a lack of support in themselves while feeling unable to do anything on their own. For any real healing to hold, the very belief of being incapable must be directly addressed in the Holistic Counseling Vis Dialogue. These cases end up being slow and need many repetitions and reminders. But if the practitioner spots this sort of belief, which the very existence of itself undermines the true healing process, then they can save many repetitions of the same cycle of empowerment, disempowerment and cut right to the chase of the underlying problem.

Whatever is blocking the case must be exposed and addressed. Address and remove obstacles to cure.

Sometimes, patients do not reveal things that are of utmost importance either because they don't think they are relevant, or they are not ready, or they simply do not think of them because it is not time for them to be revealed and addressed. I've seen this in several cases, and I am often baffled. I want to say something like, *"Uh, you could have told me that during our first appointment."* One example is of the case of the young woman in her 20s with myasthenia gravis that was not responding well to treatment. I had four appointments with her and it was on the fifth appointment where she told me something she had never shared that was the key to her whole case improving. When it was time for our appointment, I called her and she answered the phone sounding out of breath and like she was having a hard time breathing. She said she was overdue for her Mestinon and wanted to go and get it right away. I told her to wait. I said sometimes it is best to work right while you are having symptoms. Perhaps it was because she was not medicated and the acute presence of her symptoms pushed her to reveal it to me, but that day, she told me, that right before she had gotten symptoms of myasthenia gravis, something very terrible had happened to her recent ex-boyfriend. He was in a gang and she told him if he didn't leave the gang, she would leave him. Well, it turned out that he didn't leave the gang and she did leave him. Not long after that, he was killed in gang-related violence. She then had begun blaming herself, thinking, "If I had stayed with him, maybe he would not have died." She began crying deeply during that appointment, and after she had finished crying, I asked her how her breathing was, and she said it was fine. She had the chance to observe the immediate healing effects of releasing all that grief and guilt that had led to her illness. She saw that she didn't in fact need the Mestinon, but rather to face and deal with the root cause of her illness, which she had, for some reason, waited to mention during our earlier appointments. Upon reflection, I believe it was because she was not taking her Mestinon and her symptoms were so acute that they led directly to the cause of the disease. This is an important point to take note of when working with patients that are on drugs who are not progressing. A slow, responsible removal of the drug or drugs is often necessary to be able to get a patient to heal at the root of their illness.

If you are searching for a reason a case is not advancing and you are investigating with the patient, you may need to simply ask, *"Is there something else that is important that you are not telling me, or, that you have forgotten to tell me?"* Sometimes patients 'blank out' and simply cannot remember during the appointment, but it will come up after the appointment or in a subsequent follow-up. I also tell patients they can email me if they remember something very important following an appointment.

Part IV

Additional Important Elements of Holistic Counseling

Chapter 33

Homework for the Patient

Giving Homework is a good way to ensure that the healing work will continue and the person won't just walk back into forgetting. Mindfulness is an important part of any path, whether it be spiritual or healing, and so giving patients the task of being mindful is very helpful.

I find one of the best ways to do so is through journaling. I tell a patient to keep a journal and to work through their feelings and thoughts that way. Also, I ask patients to keep a journal of their other symptoms. Which ones are getting better, which are worse? This is very helpful when assessing homeopathic remedies. I also like to ask patients to keep a dream journal. All of this can be done in one journal.

I email most patients the notes from our sessions that I have typed up to read over and refresh their memory concerning what we had exposed on a previous appointment. This is a very effective form of homework for the patient.

I also recommend movies and books to read. Sometimes a theme is so strong in a person's life, watching a movie or reading a book that deals well with that theme can bring more awareness to the patient.

I like to recommend art therapy. Painting, drawing, forming one's feelings on the canvas, or in clay, can be very moving for a patient and helps to move the water medium, connecting mind with body.

The idea is being mindful. Putting time, focus, and attention on their issues. I can tell a patient to be mindful and they will apply that practice and improve with it. Other people do not comply. It really depends on the person.

Sometimes, I will leave the patient with a custom piece of

homework or a specialized task to accomplish. For example, I had a case of a woman whose problems all boiled down to a lack of desire to take any responsibility in her life. Through investigation, it became clear that she was carrying unnecessary responsibility, and as I wrote in Chapter 19 on *No Room for Any More – Sympathetic Resonance* – the unhealthy responsibility was causing her to have no more room for what she needed to be responsible for. I gave her the task of writing all the things she was responsible for, that were healthy, and all the things she was not responsible for that she was trying to be responsible for (unhealthy). Such homework is not necessary if the patient makes a shift into a new space or a new choice and has committed to that. In this case, however, she simply did not want to take any responsibility, because of the unhealthy responsibility she was carrying, and the case was left at that, so this was a helpful exercise to get her shifting away from the unhealthy and into the healthy responsibility.

In another case of a woman with myasthenia gravis, she had some very strong issues around male-female imbalances. She had grown up believing in quite a few things about both the male and the female inside of her which were not harmonious. At the end of our first appointment, I gave her the following exercise:

Step 1 – Make a list of all characteristics that you believe about the male and female.

Step 2 – Decide which characteristics are healthy for you and which characteristics are true about the female and male (each respectively). Also, decide which characteristics are unhealthy for you and untrue about both the female and male (respectively).

Step 3 – What is keeping you, if anything at all, from being the healthy characteristic if you are not being so? And what is keeping you from stopping the unhealthy characteristics – and making such changes a reality in your life?

In another case, also of myasthenia gravis, a young woman's problem was based in the belief that she was dependent on others because she was weak. This had manifested as weakness in her body. The end of the case went as follows:

"What can you do about this feeling of weakness you have inside of you?"

"I don't know. Change my mindset."

"What would you change?"

"My mindset of having to depend on someone emotionally. Or having the need to have someone fill up for my emotional needs."

"Do you think you can do this?"

"Yeah."

I offered the following exercise to do at home:

If you notice you're feeling incapable or dependent or very weak, then just be aware of that.

Step 1 is just being aware.

Step 2 is acceptance of the fact that this is how you feel. Give yourself a break. Being graceful with yourself.

Step 3 is to change your mindset about this – that you are emotionally dependent and weak.

I then worked with her on a statement of letting go and then positive statements to replace the space where there was the negative.

Step 3a "I let go of the idea that I need others to fill up my emotional needs."

Step 3b "I am able to think more rationally and being able to see the good in everything so I won't be overly emotional and I will stop myself from reacting too much."

I then asked her: *"How do you say that more simply?"*

She replied, "I am emotionally independent and I can think rationally when it is necessary."

In this case, working on the exercise, the patient actually had an aha moment and a shift in her awarness. She said:

"That is so good. Makes so much sense. I have needed others to fill up my emotional needs."

I also work with an exercise that I developed, which is quite like this last exercise. It's called the *Present, Past, Future Exercise.* This is a great exercise to offer as homework. Doing it once or twice every day gives a time to focus on releasing and replacing the belief system.

The Present – Past – Future Exercise

With a patient, work on the precise language of the belief system to be released. For example, the belief is that "I am not good enough." Make sure they feel it is accurate. Then do part 1.

Part 1 – Say, "I let go of the "belief"" in the present tense.

I let go of the idea that I am not good enough. I let go of the idea that I am not good enough.

I let go of the idea that I am not good enough. I let go of the idea that I am not good enough.

(I let go as in I am now, presently, letting go.)

Keep saying it for 36 seconds in the present tense. Do not let any thoughts distract you or cause the mind to wander.

Then take a breather for a few seconds, and move on to part 2.

Part 2 – Saying I let go of the "belief" in the past tense.

So in part 1, we were literally saying it as if it was happening in the present tense. Now, the words stay the same, but the intention shifts to the idea that we have already done so, and so we say:

I let go of the idea that I am not good enough. I let go of the idea that I am not good enough.

I let go of the idea that I am not good enough. I let go of the idea that I am not good enough.

(I let go, as in I already have let go.)

Do it for 36 seconds without distraction or mind-drifting.

Part 3 – Selecting a new empowered, healthy thought that is true to the self and aligned with who the person wants to be (their sense of I AM) – This is the future part.

Work with the patient on choosing a corresponding thought that is truer to themselves than the false belief. Get the language precise and to the point that feels good to the patient.

I am good enough. I am worthy. I am ok.

I am good enough. I am worthy. I am ok.

Say it for 36 seconds with full concentration. No distractions. That is it for the whole exercise.

If done right, this exercise can be extremely helpful and only takes 108 seconds, i.e less than 2 minutes, which is about the attention span of many people in our modern smart-phone technological age.

With all and any exercise like this, as well as with the release of any belief system, it is important to remember the Buddhist tenet – The thought becomes the word becomes the deed becomes the habit becomes the character. Recognition is a great start to begin the change in beliefs. The thought – I am good enough. I know I am. Next comes the word. Speaking the new truth out loud. Saying it to the self and others. "I am good enough." But only when the action is carried out that is representative of the new belief will there be true healing. So a person can think and say all that they want concerning the healing of a belief and the implantation of the new and healthy thought, but if they do not take the step to act accordingly, then the healing has not fully taken place. For example, with the belief "I am not good enough," a person may have the tendency to short change themselves in what they are worthy of, possibly in a job position, in a relationship, in terms of how much income they can make, how they allow others to speak to them, etc. If the belief is changed but the person does nothing to change how the life is set up around the old belief, they will not fully recover and be healed. It is when they seek a better job position, accept a better salary for themselves, choose a partner more suitable for them, and not allow others to treat them in an unkind fashion that they will truly begin to heal. Because how deep can a healing be if a person is still behaving the way they were with the old belief? So the action and subsequent change of life is important to see. Telling this to patients as part of their homework is also a good idea.

Chapter 34

What to Do during Follow-Ups

Approaching follow-ups is quite simple. How is the patient doing? That's the basic premise. Each follow-up is almost like a brand new start and after checking into how the items and issues that arose during the previous appointment are explored, one should jump into the case as if seeing it for the first time.

After each case, I summarize the key points, issues, themes, and beliefs that arose during the dialogue. This is what an example of a summary of key points would look like to me following a case.

Key Core Themes of the Case

Responsibility – fear of it, avoidance – too responsible. Very young responsibility.

Reversal of roles – 'I am the only rational one in my family.' Therefore I am responsible for everyone.

Delusion of being incapable.

Lack of being supported.

Not moving forward. Stuckness.

Anger – towards self over being incapable.

Restless foot with anxiety and laughter.

Grief with guilt.

Feeling of floating.

Then, before a follow-up, I will review each of these key points so that I can ask how the patient is doing in regards to each symptom. This is quite similar to homeopathic follow-ups after administering a remedy to the patient. We want to know if the issues that were a problem for the patient are still a problem. If, for instance, four out of five issues from the previous session are no longer an issue, and only one is, then congratulate the person on the four that have been resolved and proceed to ask them what is still troubling them about the fifth, unresolved issue. This will open up the dialogue and take off where they left off.

I also start off the follow-up appointment with a simple question, "How are you doing?" and take it from there, only to inquire later about the specific issues and beliefs that arose the last appointment.

If a patient says, "I am doing terribly bad." Ask them to explain what is happening, but make sure to inquire when, precisely, they began to feel bad. It is surprising how "in the moment" a patient can be, forgetting the three or four weeks prior to the present appointment when they were feeling very well. Now, perhaps for the last few days they slipped back into feeling bad, and they won't express it as, "I was doing so well and now I am not anymore." Many, if not, most patients will make it sound like they're no better. It's just that they have forgotten the 3-4 weeks of improvement.

If they say they were doing well for a certain amount of time and then they began to feel bad again, that is a great opportunity to explore *what exactly happened* to trigger them, push them off course, or cause them to relapse. This may simply be a return to the very "Rome" that you had arrived at during the previous consultation and the patient simply is unaware of it on a conscious level.

In a previous dialogue, you may have unearthed many avenues that could have been explored but were not. It is during the follow-ups that you can explore such avenues. It will be helpful to keep good notes like, "To be explored – how he feels about his uncle." Or, "To be explored –issues regarding money." If one of these unaddressed issues is an avenue that truly has a crucial issue that needs to be addressed, in a follow-up, the patient will most likely reveal this, based in the fact that it is troubling them and leading to struggle and suffering. So, it is at this time, during a follow-up, when the avenue that could have been explored and was not, is addressed. If the practitioner takes good notes during a previous appointment, even if the patient does not spontaneously bring up a subject by themselves during the follow-up, the practitioner can inquire about an avenue that was opened up that did not necessarily seem resolved by the "Rome" of the last session.

"Last appointment you had mentioned briefly your issues regarding money. Can we talk about that now?" or, *"Last time, it seemed as if there was some issue regarding your uncle. Is that something you feel you'd like to discuss at this time?"*

I schedule my follow-ups six weeks apart. This is because I work both with Holistic Counseling and homeopathy and like to give the remedy and the changes in consciousness a good chance to work, make changes in the Vital Force, and give time to see what is left to address. Things in Nature take time to unfold. If the follow-ups are too frequent, it's like we keep putting on a new layer of paint before the previous layer has dried. If I were only offering Holistic Counseling, six weeks would probably be a little too long in between appointments. I definitely feel weekly visits are too frequent, and even one appointment every two weeks may be a little too frequent, since it does take time for a patient to integrate the lessons learned during a previous appointment. Also, a person needs time in their life to make the changes that they learned they must implement. If the follow-ups are too frequent, the patient goes into a perpetual "learning and healing" mode, without the required action and change they need to apply in their lives. Some patients like to do the work in the office, but not in their life. When the follow-ups are spaced adequately and seem at least a little distant in the future, the patient cannot rely strictly on the appointments to get them through their lives. They must take responsibility and take the necessary steps to create the life that they really want and/or that will result in health and happiness. Time, in such cases, is like the pressure cooker that pushes them to take action. Then again, if the follow-ups are too distant, their memory of what is most important that was learned during the previous appointment can fade and leave the patient to revert back to a former and habitual state of mind. I think follow-ups every 3-4 weeks for strictly Holistic Counseling would be ideal. Once every two weeks is possible for cases that are currently in high degrees of suffering and confusion. I would leave weekly appointments only to patients in dire straits, where they need regular and closely spaced visits in order to gain some ground on the powerful force of the illness that has come to inhabit their being.

The goal of every dialogue is to have a big release, a getting down to "Rome" and then helping the patient choose a new way of being. It happens during most appointments, but not all the time. If it doesn't, I offer homework, exercises, like journaling, mindfulness, meditation, and send them off with a homeopathic remedy. I have found that most of my follow-ups run for about one hour to one hour and fifteen minutes in order to have a big release and a shift. It takes time to get back into the thick of things with people. I often go one and a half hours and so normally book my follow-ups accordingly. On rare occasions, I even go to 2 hours during a follow-up. At times the follow-ups will last for one half hour to fourty-five minutes.

Sometimes, the follow-up is a return to the original "Rome." I described a few cases where this continued to happen. Eventually, it began to stick, but it seems that some patients need reminders, in the sense that, they get lost back into the unconsciousness of their life, and they forget. Then the waters of doubt will get cleared once again during the follow-up and they remember, only to forget again. Each person is different and some may require only one parting of the waters of doubt to be in total awareness, and others require several visits beyond their "Rome" to get accustomed to being there.

In other cases, the follow-up brings a continuation down through the Rabbit Hole, to deeper and deeper places in the person's life that represent older wounds and their accompanying false beliefs that are embedded further and further back in time. It is a path that can seem to go on forever. And it truly may take a lifetime, but the path of healing is not an infinite one. Yes, spiritual growth and learning about who we are is an infinite path, where one can always continue to grow further from the point one finds oneself. But the healing of wounds and false beliefs of the past is finite, because those beliefs are false, and that which is false is not infinite. Only that which is true is infinite, so the path of illness, as it rests on false ideas, does come to an end. Thank goodness!

Chapter 35

Additional Important Miscellaneous Elements to Consider During the Vis Dialogue

Each bullet point (•) seen in this chapter deals with a stand-alone additional insight into the Holistic Counseling process.

• Check into the feelings

Because the Vis Dialogue is largely an intellectual process in that it involves questions, it's a good idea to have a patient check into their feelings during a dialogue. I'll often ask, *"What are you feeling right now?"* just to remind the patient to check in with their feelings, and to connect mind with emotion, so that the watery medium helps bridge between the mind and the body.

• Don't follow empty answers

If you ask a question and you can tell that the patient has not answered the question and has not gone anywhere, don't follow their response. It will only be a waste of time. This occurs when you can really sense a momentum and there is a keen feeling of "getting somewhere." Then, when you ask another question, there is a loss of momentum in their response as if the patient "dropped the ball." In order to preserve the momentum and continue along toward the deeper, more important direction of "getting somewhere," ignore their response and ask another question. It can be the same question asked exactly in the same way, or in a slightly different way, or from a different angle.

• Technique of retracing the steps up and out of the Rabbit Hole

We have spoken quite a bit about going into and down the Rabbit Hole. A very valuable technique is retracing the patient's footsteps back UP the Rabbit Hole, to clarify the connection between where they started and where they arrived. It's a form of feedback that goes through the reverse order of steps that allowed one to go from A to Z. A patient can get so deeply immersed in the Vis Dialogue that they may even forget their original complaint, or the way they initially expressed it. To retrace their footsteps reminds them of where they started and then the steps and connections made from the start to the bottom line belief. It can create quite a "click" in their minds. "This underlying belief where we concluded is related to my issue that I started with?!?! Wow!" It's sometimes hard to believe that the bottom is related to the top. That is why, by retracing each step backward and up and out of the Rabbit Hole, it is something undeniable because each step is retraced. Using some form of note taking is helpful and for many practitioners, would be necessary, unless you have a great memory that you can operate backwards. The practitioner does not need to highlight *each* and *every single* step that had been taken, but rather, can highlight the key points and steps along the way.

Recall the case of the woman whose boyfriend made her feel stupid in Chapter 29 in the part about *Reflecting Elsewhere* questions. We ended up at an event where the patient, at the age of 5 or 6 years old, thought that she had angered her father and it was going to result in him leaving the family and it was all her fault. At this point, I had given some feedback, which actually does involve retracing steps up and out of the Rabbit Hole. In essence, feedback is often a look back up and out of the Rabbit hole, though normally, for only a step or two back at a time. However, this feedback I had given was for several steps of awareness and it did serve to bridge a bottom line awareness with the starting point. The most effective way to use this technique is not only to make the steps backward and up and out of the Rabbit hole, but to equally make the connections for the patient, as in the feedback + technique.

"So making your father angry caused him to storm out of the house. You thought that he would never come back. This brought up the worst feeling for you, which you will do anything to avoid, including making yourself small and stupid so you don't make anyone angry with you. Is that about right?"
She said yes. That was a very important connection that helped her see how her present complaint of feeling stupid was related to the fear that she had angered her father. In another case of a woman with diabetes, there was a clear string of connections between where we began at the beginning discussing her diabetes and where we ended with her feeling and belief that she didn't matter. When we got down to the bottom line, which was underlying everything for her, I asked her if she saw the connection between how "I don't matter" connected back to her diabetes. And she said, "No," she didn't see the connection. So I traced it up "Out of the Rabbit Hole" for her so that she could make the connection. Here's what I said, *"Because you feel you don't matter, you do everything you can to make yourself feel like you do matter to others, which includes taking on twice the work and feeling responsible for everyone and doing everything for others. It is during times when you've taken on so much responsibility that feels so heavy to you that you have gained a lot of weight. When you gain weight, your diabetes goes up. Can you see the connection now?"*
She said, "Yes!"
This case was also very interesting because it truly appeared that the patient would gain weight during times when she wasn't eating that much and was controlling her caloric intake. It was just due to her working extra hard to matter to everyone that she gained weight. It struck me that because of her very strong feeling that she didn't matter, she was compensating by trying to "matter." The feeling of someone who doesn't "matter" is that they are unimportant and also insubstantial. Literally, the word "matter" here applied to her feeling like she had no matter, no

earthly substance. I believe her compensation of needing to feel like she mattered added weight to her body to give her a more tangible sense of having some substantial solidness to her – more "matter."

• *Choose to engage*

Every case, every time, every follow-up, make the choice to engage with the patient again. Don't sit back and expect the dialogue to deepen without the clear intention to help them to go deeper. There is inertia; both in the patient and the practitioner. If you do not make a clear commitment to helping the person go deeper, you may be choosing to not engage and this will not help a patient to dig deeper. Upon each follow-up, it is amazing to what extent one can further deepen awareness toward the root of the person's problems. But that does require a full engagement. And it must be present in the heart of the practitioner. So choose to engage during every appointment.

• *Be like a hunter*

During the Vis Dialogue, a good attitude to have is the idea of being like a hunter when getting close to the "kill." I realize this is quite a violent metaphor, but bear with me. Like a tiger, once you get a whiff of the bottom line, and you know you're close to *closing the deal*, don't stop until you see the person break free. It's a kind of relentless focus and hunt to help a person break through. It is not being controlling, per se, yet it is related to being very engaged and not allowing a patient to wriggle out of taking the last steps toward change. If a tiger gets close to their prey and they relax right before they attain their goal, the prey can get away. This is especially important in light of the fact that when a patient gets close to change, the illness can rise up to oppose the change. So the practitioner must hold a sort of energetic intensity and focus to help a patient not escape right at the end, despite them seeking healing. They are locked in the headlights of your questions and you are not turning those headlights off until they break free. Do not "let go" or relax one's focus too much to let the prey slip away while one is close to the end.

• *Looking for connected not disconnected responses*
At times, you will notice a person is answering as if all of their energy and awareness is entirely up in their heads, and they are theorizing about themselves, rather than connectedly responding. At such a time say, *"Ok, can you just take a moment and connect with the feeling and sense you have in your body about what we're talking about?"* This will help a person connect to the beliefs and feelings that are actually a part of their problem rather than any disconnected theory about what's going on. It will save a lot of time. It's ok to have people that are very intellectual respond to their answers through the mental sphere. But sometimes people have told themselves stories about who they are and how life is for such a long time that it's difficult to get them to connect to what they're really believing, feeling emotionally and physically. So sometimes a practitioner has to help get into the Rabbit Hole by helping them engage more where the issues live in the body. That is then connected to the emotional and mental realms of struggles that are not in harmony with their I AM statements and so it is the correct path to explore; the path that is connected to the pain and suffering, not the stories in their head they've told themselves to avoid dealing with their pain. Only follow connected responses.

• *Nothing beneath the Foundation*
Consider the basement floor is the last level of the house of cards. There's nothing beyond that, which means that the basement floor is the foundation, the last underlying belief that is holding up the rest of the House of Cards. Just recognizing this can be very freeing. Like with the question I was asked that essentially

burst the bubble of my illness, "What makes you think you need to be perfect?" I could see that there was nothing that supported this idea. There was no deeper belief that the idea of needing to be perfect stood on. When I opened the door to gaze down the stairs to the lower level, there were no stairs and no lower level. Empty space. Void. Nothingness. Seeing this can really help a patient pop a hole in the inflated belief. Before they see past the basement floor, their belief is inflated with intensity and the "realness of it" seems powerful and commands obeisance. But when a patient recognizes there is nothing else deeper, and that there is nothing that "holds up" the belief, it can begin to immediately dissolve. It did with me and I have seen this have a huge impact in peoples' lives when they get to the basement floor and there's nothing else. It is amazing to ask a line of questions and to arrive at an answer where there is no more stream to follow.

"What makes you think that everything depends on you?"

"I don't know. I can see that this is silly. I never thought of this before, but it is not true."

It's as if the person continued to allow the foundation of their house of cards to stand solid because it was just one or two steps beyond the full awareness of their conscious minds. When the torch is allowed to light up that level of thinking, it does not hold up. There is no fight. It just has never been addressed or explored so closely before. The foundation, where it may have seemed like it was made out of stone, is made out of flimsy cobwebs that are easily brushed away or burned away with the torch of exploration.

This happens often enough that it makes me marvel at how ready some people are to let go of their beliefs. Even consciously aware and living in just the very next level higher in the House of Cards, the lower foundation can stand strong. But with one level deeper of simple exploration, the seeming reality of the lowest belief crumbles to the ground and everything else that was standing on it falls with it.

When this happens, by going back over the line of questions that led to that point with the patient, we can then see that everything that stood upon the belief with no foundation, no basis, can also be released.

• *The Healing Power of Nature continues to do its work, even following the appointment*

At times during dialogues, we're unable to get as deeply as we'd like to help patients resolve their "Rome." However, don't despair. With all the deep questioning, The Healing Power of Nature gets stirred up and, like a flowing tincture, inches its way into and through the cracks and crevasses of the subconscious mind. This enables the patient to make awarenesses after the appointment is over, either later during the same day, or during the days that follow.

• *"Life-time" beliefs*

There are certainly other times when some negative belief patterns that are so deeply ingrained into a person's genetic code means that it may take them a lifetime to feel and actually be free of them. Don't despair. This life, in so many countless ways is such a beautiful mystery. There can be issues of karma, reincarnation to resolve past life struggles, miasms, inheritance of core familial genetic issues, and more. It is not for the practitioner to worry about solving every problem for every patient. The gift that the practitioner can provide for the patient, and what is within our ability, is to help them, at the very least, come to a clear understanding of what the makeup of their negative belief system is all about. Even if they are unable to find the key to release themselves from this deeply ingrained negative belief system, to help provide awareness can then lead to acceptance. Even if the belief system does not change and is not released, if a person is aware of what they believe and they accept that about themselves, the level of peace augments tremendously as compared to carrying a negative belief system that a person doesn't fully grasp, comprehend, and toward which has no acceptance.

I am not saying that at times it is impossible, strictly that it can be so hard that it seems impossible to help release some negative belief systems in some patients. However, with other healing modalities, especially those that are able to move stuck energies even at the level of the genetic code, like homeopathy, then given enough time, patience, and persistence, we can help accelerate the mysterious stuckness of some of the deepest problems.

• Getting to the core belief early in the session

Don't worry if you get to a core belief early in the session. There is no need for it to take a long time to develop. You can launch into the *Transition* and *Closing questions* right away. The reason why this is ok, is that A) If the belief that is encountered early in session is the core belief, why not address it early if it is clear? Why not move in the direction of cure right away? Sometimes the *Transition* and *Closing questions* can take a long time, so you'll have more time to give them room. B) If it is not the deepest core belief, when asked the *Closing question*: **"Is there anything stopping you from changing this?"** the next deepest belief will naturally emerge that will open up an avenue to explore deeper down the Rabbit Hole. So *Transition* and *Closing questions* can be used early on in a session and Nature will decide how far the Rabbit Hole really goes.

• Explore the contradiction

Often in a person's story, you will hear some form of contradiction between what they are saying they want, or about who they are, and then again something later that contradicts those previous statements. For example, you hear a person complaining how people are mean to them. Everyone is treating them poorly. But then, in recounting their story, it sounds very much like, they, themselves, are mean to others as well. They won't express this openly, but anyone listening from the sidelines could pick up this contradiction. Here a little chutzpah is necessary in the feedback. I would say, *"You say that people are being mean to you and treating you poorly, and yet it sounds as if you are doing the same thing in this situation you just mentioned. What makes you do that?"* Just as Holistic Counseling works so well by going through the negative, exposing such a contradiction can really "cut to the chase" and help a person recognize how they have been operating largely from an unconscious place that is in opposition to how they really want to be. The story they have told themselves does not line up with the reality of how they are really being. Such contradictions are also very valuable in homeopathy, as they represent focal points of pathology. This example was with a case I had where the patient responded, "I didn't realize I was even doing that. Oh my! I must be doing the very thing to others that has wounded me." Then I repeated the question, *"What makes you do that?"* The patient responded, "I am getting back at those that have done it to me." Which of course didn't make sense, because how can being mean to others that hadn't wounded her, actually get back at those who did wound her earlier in life. Speaking it out loud like this helped the patient recognize that fact. What then occurred is that the deeper, more influential pain could be addressed, because the activity that the patient had been attempting to compensate for their wound is removed.

In another case, a man in his sixties had a very strong contradiction that helped us move quickly toward the cause of his problem – self-loathing and wanting to destroy himself. The contradiction became clear after I recognized that he went through much effort to take very good care of himself, only to do something that was very harmful for his health. It was like a sabotage of all his good work. When I brought this contradiction to his attention, he said it was a pattern he had his entire life. As a younger man, he would exercise and stay in top shape and then drink himself into a deep drunken stupor afterwards, only to repeat the pattern the next day. Later in life, when he developed myasthenia gravis, he would make the utmost efforts to eat the best food, order the most promising supplements, only to beat himself up and torment himself with his failures.

The exposure of the contradiction brings to light such a large schism in a person's life that addressing it directly really helps circumvent much dialogue. My feedback was, *"On the one hand, you take care of yourself so much, yet on the other hand, it seems as if you're shooting yourself in the foot. What makes you do that?"* Clearly, he consciously wanted to be well. He did everything he could to make himself better, more than many patients I had seen. Yet his severe attack on himself belied a strong force inside of him that sought his own destruction. Upon revelation of this contradiction, he explained that he felt like he didn't deserve to live since he had not been able to help his mother, all those long years, when she was suffering from severe mental/emotional illness. How can he possibly get better, despite all his efforts, when he had this desire to destroy himself? Remember the puppy-dog body's mirroring of the attacking of the self in auto-immune illness. The contradiction helped cut right to the chase so that we could begin exploring his choices surrounding desiring to hurt himself.

Another variation of this theme of exploring the contradiction is to explore something that makes you feel very curious to know something more about it or that it did not make sense. The patient says something and it doesn't quite make sense, and you feel you need more info. This can often lead to a breakthrough into a deeper space, since they have expressed something that doesn't make sense, which means they are not expressing themselves well, which means they are out of touch. Therefore, a connection is asking to be made in the space between that poor communication where there's a disconnect that results in you, the practitioner, wanting to make sense of what they've said. Follow that instinct.

• *Let Truth be the judge for each individual in families or groups*
When working with couples, or with more than one person in a family, the practitioner's purpose is to let Truth be the judge for each individual. Allow the Vis Dialogue to unfold for each person regardless of the needs or intentions of the partner or relative of the patient you are also working with. For instance, Jack's girlfriend wants you to make Jack better so she can be with him. But in working with Jack through the Vis Dialogue, it becomes clear he doesn't want to be with her. Jack's truth guides him toward leaving the relationship even if his conscious mind and his girlfriend's will are for them to be together. As another example, when working with both spouses of a marriage, if it is revealed to one of the spouses that they need to assert themselves more, but it is known that this may upset their partner, then, Truth guides the individual, and they should therefore assert themselves more. There is a bottom line here that states – one's truth is good for oneself and for everyone else. Even if, in a person's conscious control, in their fears, they are not happy with another's truth and with another setting themselves free, that truth is nevertheless good for them as well. It makes them confront their fear, and pushes them to release their control. Evolutionarily speaking, it is good for them to have their partner being more true to themselves, even if they don't like it consciously and it makes them confront their darkness, which is something they have wanted to avoid.

• *Minor beliefs not connected to pathology vs core beliefs that are*
In some cases, we may work with the patient and help them release beliefs, thinking these are the core, but it turns out it did

not touch the core of the disease. I'd call these minor beliefs not connected to the pathology, because it is not at the root cause of the disease presently being addressed. The belief itself can still be very deeply rooted into a limitation of being that is very liberating to release. However, even with such a deep rooted belief released, the disease itself will not really improve. This is therefore a minor belief not connected to the pathology and this will become clear during a follow-up. We have to go back to the drawing board, and explore to find the core or pursue where we might have left off an unexplored channel. A core belief, that is, one that, when released, will truly help resolve an illness, is one that is wrapped up in the chief complaint. One will find elements in the pathology itself of the belief that led to it. The sensations, the language described, the restrictions caused by the pathology will all point to or reflect the core belief responsible for the disease. Also, while beginning to explore through the pathology, by asking the questions described in *Chapter 30 – Technique of going through the Physical Symptoms to Get to the Root Cause*, if you follow these questions and continue to follow the stream and go deeper into the Rabbit Hole, when you see the belief that reflects the pathology and the emotions, it will become clear that you have arrived at "Rome." You are there. If, for instance, it is not quite the bottom line of the House of Cards, when you ask, *"Do you want to keep living this way?"* and they say, "No," and then you ask, *"Is there anything stopping you from changing this?"* And they say, "Yes." wherever that leads, will likely be the deeper aspect of their case that is even more core and therefore, more fundamental. The bottom line in this bullet point is that we may explore a path with a patient and help them release a belief that appears to be at their core, but if the pathology of their disease does not improve, then that is not the deepest part of the core. It was likely necessary to clear that minor belief or issue first, in order to be able to get deeper later. So there is no harm done. It is important to follow Nature and let Nature reveal the way to heal the person. Sometimes it can take several appointments to get to the deepest choice underlying the root cause of someone's disease. We cannot rush it or project our expectations. We must truly allow Nature to reveal when the healing is complete.

- *Only the shell remains*

I've noticed with some cases, and even in my own healing, that after a while of being aware of an issue, and a pattern of false belief, working on it, journaling about it, and maintaining focus and awareness about it to resolve and release it, all that remains is an empty shell of the issue. It is as if the flakey skin of the snake remains as a wisp and it has no more substance than that. A person, with this shell, can be under the impression that they still have the issue, but truly, for all intents and purposes, it is gone. The only thing left of the old belief and pattern is the *memory* and the *habit* of being accustomed to its presence, but the choice has no more charge and no power. All that remains is to make the choice to change into a new, happier pattern and then to act on the change. I had a case of a man who had struggled with a lot of lust in his life. He had felt so subject to the whim of his desire for women that he didn't feel in control of himself. He only realized he was out of control and couldn't stop, when he tried to stop because it was causing him to often lose his focus, his center, and become highly distracted whenever a woman was around that he found attractive. When we did the Vis Dialogue about it, we uncovered that it had a lot to do with the patterns he had been fed growing up when he was around other guys. You were cool if you slept with a lot of girls. The prettier, the more status it represented and the more respect. Desiring respect was a form of compensation for him because he had not felt respected by his father. So he discovered this and decided he did not wish to continue having to "get women" to make up for his father being undemonstrative and withholding support and respect toward him when he was a child. As we continued to work together, he would tell me that it wasn't really getting any better. He still would have to look at every woman that walked by to see if she was "hot" as a continuation of his addictive compensatory pattern. We continued to work together on this issue and "chip away" at it. Then, one day during a dialogue, he said the following: "I find myself still looking at women, as if I desire them. But there is no pull there. It's like I don't even care. I have no feeling about it, just that I am still looking at them." This is a tell-tale sign that the pattern has nothing but the shell of the habit still there. So then he realized that all that was left was for him to actually stop looking at every woman walking by was to do just that, stop. That is the action that reflects the final step of the healing process. Once he began to do just that, there was nothing drawing him and in time, the pattern went away, except for the occasional peek here and there, which in any other person, is natural and fine. But for him, it was about getting back his choice in the matter. He felt much more in control of how he wanted to be and not subject to his desires, and underlying wounds.

In other cases, this can look like exploring a belief and realizing there is nothing there holding the person back from releasing it. No more emotional charge. No bodily reflection. Just the old habit that remains. Explaining this to a patient can be helpful. I've gone through patterns with patients that reveal these empty shells. When we explore how they feel about it and what is holding them back from changing it, there is actually nothing. So all that is left is making the choice to stop acting out, in whatever way it is they are acting out that supports the remaining shell.

Some unhealthy patterns and wounds are so deep that they may take a very long time, even a lifetime, to resolve. It is especially in these protracted struggles we have with our wounds where only the shell may remain, and due to such a long battle, there is nothing left but to recognize that the pattern has changed. There's nothing of substance holding the person back from total resolution of the life-long belief. It's good to illustrate this to a patient when you recognize it may be the case and encourage them to act as if the issue is already gone.

• *When does the healing end?*

The answer: It depends. There are two ways of looking at healing. One – is healing the human condition. Two – for a particular illness.

One – For the Human Condition, the healing never ends. We are born in separation. It is a root of all potential for the struggles and illnesses we face in this world. This may be likened to the very root of Psora, that miasm in homeopathic philosophy which is primary and acts as the root "terrain" for all chronic illness. It is the state of having free will, of believing there is even a choice for separation between ourselves and Creation. If one were to master this separation and achieved a state of Oneness, one could say the healing of the separation ended, and so would begin the next state of evolution of the soul. One can say that the healing of the Human Condition ends, and the Avatar/Ascended Master evolutionary process begins. However, the state of Avatar is part of the Human Condition, so the healing, in truth, does not end; it just takes on different challenges and requirements. From there, the Avatar/Ascended Master could ascend into a higher state of existence, even closer to the Creator. From that point, there is continual growth and evolution.

Healing, therefore, is truly a form of evolution and a form of return to the primary source of the Creator. It must happen in steps, otherwise, if a soul was to be catapulted back to the prime Source of their Being without going through an acclimatization and adjustment to each level of proximity and power, they would burn up in the intensity of the fire and the brilliance of the Light.

For healing and expansion of the boundaries of the human

condition, it requires a soul to explore all forms of belief, even those that are taken for granted by the collective of humanity, such as the idea of separation itself. Beliefs about what is possible for a human being to achieve, to be, to witness, to feel, to explore. Beliefs such as lifespan, limitations of healing abilities, potential of human consciousness, need all be challenged for the continual evolution of the human being toward their truest and most aligned state of the soul.

Two – A particular illness does have a delineated and finite amount of healing before it is resolved. A particular illness has become condensed and crystallized through the mind-emotions and then body of a particular belief and woundedness. By addressing and clearing the root cause of that particular illness, the illness ends. So healing only takes so long as the root cause of disease is cleared and the mind, emotions, and body's state returns to harmony. Sometimes this lasts a few years, sometimes a few months, and in other cases, it can last an entire lifetime. Some cases of physical illness are actually connected to a larger collective and the person's disease is a karmic or collective endeavor of healing. The process of healing such an illness would be much longer than an illness that is delineated due to a person not being true to their I AM.

- *Part of me knows, but the other part of me doesn't feel it*
When a patient expresses that they understand they have to change and let go of a belief system, but a part of them doesn't want to, doesn't feel like it, or doesn't know if it can, then ask:

"What part of you doesn't want to?" or, *"What part of you doesn't feel like it?"* or, *"What part of you doesn't know if you can?"*

Even when people say, "A part of me" they are still speaking of themselves, so use questions to explore and investigate "the part" of them that is not on board with change. Essentially, that is just an aspect of themselves that is not on board for the healing and change. Then, following those initial questions, ask accompanying questions as you would in a regular Vis Dialogue without referring to the part, but just to the person themselves. The part then becomes integrated into the whole. For example:

"What part of you doesn't want to?"

"The part that is afraid."

"What is that part afraid of?"

"Failure."

"What is it that you are afraid of?" (Notice here how I switched from the part to you. That helps with integration.)

As another example,

"What part of you doesn't feel like changing?"

"The part of me that is lazy."

"What about changing your belief does the lazy part of you not feel like doing?"

"It seems like a lot of work."

"And so, what if it is a lot of work?"

"Then that part of me doesn't want to do it."

"What about doing a lot of work do you not want to do?"

"Well, things should just be able to go really easy, without a lot of work."

"Where did you get that idea?" Or, *"What makes you believe that things should go really easy without a lot of work?"*

"I don't know. I guess I never thought of it."

"Do you think that is something that is serving you well right now?"

"No. I guess not. It's not very helpful in light of the fact that I know some things do take hard work."

"So do you want to keep believing that things should be easy?"

"No." (A short pause here.)

"So how do you feel about changing the core belief we arrived at earlier?"

"Better. I think I can do that now."
"Great!"

• *Let go of desire*

Many mystical and spiritual traditions teach to let go of desire. And I have found this to be most true. Desire leads to suffering. But what kind of desire? The answer reminds one of the *Two Paths* metaphor. A desire or wish that comes from the heart which is aligned with the patient's I AM is healthy and good. It will often be experienced and carried out seamlessly and effortlessly, like a "no brainer." It nurtures and feels right, like an extension of the self in the moment. The other kind of desire attached to the second path, like a wool blanket, gets all sorts of things attached to it, like need, worry, anxiety, fear, stress, hatred, resentment. This becomes very heavy and taxing over time and is associated with disease. This sort of desire is based in the idea that, "I need that 'thing' or 'status' or 'whatever' to be ok." That is what leads to the suffering, because they are saying, "I am not ok without it." Such an idea makes one a slave to the desire. There is no freedom in that. If a person was to give up all of their desires of this nature, they would achieve a great amount of health, peace, and joy. This is not to say that they do nothing and sit in the grayness of neutral being. It means that they recognize and have released all desires that have a fundamental inherent belief that "I am not ok without the object that I desire." During the Vis Dialogue, you will notice where a person is attached to an unhealthy desire. It will become clear that this desire is of the kind that is like a bottomless pit. It may be easily identifiable as connected to the second path and their compensation. When you recognize this, it becomes an "opening" into the Rabbit Hole *through the negative,* because it is, in and of itself, of the nature of ego and separation unaligned with the health and well-being of the true I AM.

• *More on the path of the heart from the Two Paths metaphor*

Sometimes it can be very subtle and very difficult to decide what one's true path is. It can be a very painful path to follow one's heart. Fears need to be addressed. Friends and family members can disagree and abandon us. The New Age idea of everything should feel good, and positive, and happy can be a detriment to walking one's true path since it can often be quite difficult at first to initiate one's true call. But it is a pain that leads to growth of the Soul and will result in peace and the depth of being. The notion of "always do what you want" that is often encountered in today's self-help and New Age books can also lead to confusion because sometimes the Universe provides us not with what we outwardly think we want (path of compensation), but what we *need* to walk the path of the heart. The path of heart is the path of Love and to be oneself is to be Love. They are one and the same because our Creator is Love. Love is not always easy. Pregnancy isn't easy, neither is birth, but look at the great miracle that is born following the trials of pregnancy and labor.

• *Just Be*

Sometimes, after all the pondering and talk and questions and answers, you just gotta be.

Chapter 36

The Limitations of Holistic Counseling

What are the Limitations of Holistic Counseling?

Despite Holistic Counseling being such a wonderful gift to help people, and ourselves, heal, there are certain situations and types of patients that do limit how much we can help someone. It may be in part due to where our society is at the present and the incorrect expectations people have to not take any responsibility for their health and rely on the doctor to do all the work. It may also be due to our own issues that get in the way of being unbiased, uncontrolling, and sensitive enough to help the tough cases that may trigger us. At times, we cannot use Holistic Counseling at all.

Here are some of the limitations of Holistic Counseling. Please make sure to not allow these to become a belief-system in and of themselves, like a knee-jerk reaction to deem the case unworkable because it fits one of these criteria. Besides the first point on this list, there are really no situations, as a general rule, that are impossible to help, at least to some degree.

• **Unconscious.**
For obvious reasons.

• **Not wanting to be there. No permission.**
When the spouse sends her husband, and he doesn't want to be there, it will be a clumsy dance that has no beauty and no reward to attempt to Holistically Counsel the husband, unless he changes his mind for himself, and decides he wants to get something out of it for himself. So make sure the patient wants to be there for themselves.

• **Drugs.**

This is a limitation that definitely varies in the degree that it affects one's ability to help their patients. In some cases, a person's drugs are a straightjacket on their system, holding the symptoms in check and not allowing anything to move either backward, into a worsening of symptoms, or forward, into resolution and healing. I've seen this with many cases, especially those drugs which affect the mind like antidepressants, and anxiolytics, and other drugs that have global effects on a person's entire body like steroids. With antidepressants, it's like the person is blanked out in their mind when it comes down to a certain depth. They are not quite there. They are out of touch with themselves and do not know how to respond to questions like, "How does it feel?" or, "Where did this come from?" Often people are very reliant on their drugs and are afraid to return to where they were before they went on the drugs – depressed, afraid, anxious, feeling out of control, etc. In such a case, if you are hitting a wall with the patient that is due to their drug, and they are unwilling to slowly and responsibly come off their drug, that is a limitation of Holistic Counseling and holistic healing in general, for that matter. I tell the patient that the drug is straight-jacketing their system and ask them if they are willing to come off it. Some say yes, others no. When a patient says no, then I work with other modalities, mostly homeopathy, to help them feel stronger and hopefully ready to come off their drugs. I'll also explain that the drug is just suppressing symptoms and the root cause of their issues is not going away and in fact, may be getting worse over time, due to the suppression. In cases of severe pathology, the coming off of drugs has to be navigated with the utmost care and with follow-ups planned strategically to deal with any worsening of symptoms that may arise.

In other cases, a person can be on one or several drugs and the drugs are not really doing much anyway, so the Holistic Counseling can penetrate right down to where it needs to be to help the patient. When a patient feels better and the portion of the mind that was locked up that led to the illness is freed, then they feel more confident and able to come off their drugs.

• **Very advanced, destructive pathology**

> Such chronic supposed-to-be-incurable disease as tubercu-losis, cancer, locomotor ataxia, paresis, paralysis agitans, infantile paralysis, secondary and tertiary syphilis, etc., yield to the natural treatments, provided there is enough vitality in the system to respond to treatment and the destruction of vital parts and organs has not too far advanced. Henry Lindlahr (1862 – 1924)

If a person has multiple sclerosis with advanced demyelination of their nerves, it is much less likely to be able to help their physical symptoms than if the healing had begun right in the beginning of the case. This is not to say that no healing can happen, because mental and emotional healing can occur, so that the cause that had led to the illness is cleared, the person is more enlightened about themselves, and has a deeper understanding. Normally, when this is the case a certain wisdom also emerges in the patient, and there is a greater acceptance of their situation so they are not raging against it. Emphysema, cirrhosis of the liver, osteoarthritis, and other destructive processes in the body where the body tissue has been damaged beyond repair may be impos-sible to help with holism. I say may be impossible because I do also believe in healing that defies the logic of our present under-standing of the body. There have been advanced cases of MS that have been cured. Cases of osteoarthritis, where it is bone on bone and there is no more cartilage even present in the joint, have improved during healing with certain modalities. So nothing is impossible and miracles do occur.

- **Children – young children, babies, preverbal**

Obviously, preverbal and very young babies and children cannot be holistically counseled. However, when a child can do Holistic Counseling depends on the child as an individual and not on the age, as a general rule. I've seen very young children ages four or five able to answer some simple questions with surprising awareness. Others gloss over and do not understand the meaning whatsoever. The practitioner can try a few questions on the child to see if they are ready for such a dialogue. You may be surprised. You may also be surprised to find that some teenagers are unable, or perhaps unwilling, to closely consider and answer the questions of the Vis Dialogue and seem more intent on staring with an absent or annoyed look on their faces.

- **Very elderly**

Some elderly people do very well with Holistic Counseling, whereas others are just too fixed in their mindset, too wanting to be taken care of, too indoctrinated in the allopathic model of medicine, and at times, on too many drugs to be able to make any movement on the holistic level. Also, sometimes, it is a combination of two or more factors that make it very hard to help them change their views on life. What we can say is that the Caboose of disease has a lot of momentum in the body, and depending on how long the patient has been sick, there can also be a lot of momentum in the mental and emotional spheres due to the habit of having the disease or belief for so long. This really varies from case to case and the practitioner must work on an individual level, and not pass a sweeping judgment over the elderly population. Some may be too stuck at seventy years old, whereas, others, in their nineties, may show great promise and readiness to change.

- **Mental/emotional illness**

When a patient has severe schizophrenia, it is not possible to help them with Holistic Counseling. However, more mild cases can respond well. When problems are caught in their early stages, no matter what the situation, there is always a greater degree of motility in the mind than later. The mind does get used to the situation and being outside of it seems less likely, the longer the condition has continued. Bipolar cases are less likely to respond in any constructive way to any questions during the manic phase, but in the depressive phase, there is a greater chance to get real answers and to have an impact. When a person is severely mentally ill, you cannot help them, because the very tool with which we heal, i.e. the mind, is not in a state that is available for the healing.

When a person is so extremely emotional, perhaps hysterical or really so stuck in the emotion that they do not want to do any mental activity, they will not respond to Holistic Counseling. Later, perhaps some time later, or following a good remedy, they will be more able.

• **Language barrier**
When there is a language barrier between practitioner and patient, Holistic Counseling won't work. The language must be strong enough between patient and doctor that at least some of the subtler aspects of the language are grasped.

• **Third World/Developing countries**
I was in Nigeria and tried to do Holistic Counseling with some of the patients I saw there. It didn't work. Some people are just subsisting on the very basics of life. They have little self-reflection. Sitting in reflection and meditation is a luxury in life that not all people have had the chance to do. Given other life circumstances, those very same people could benefit greatly from the Vis Dialogue, but life for them is strongly about surviving day by day and there is not a lot of questioning of circumstance. They live largely in the body, and in the emotions, and not a great

deal in the intellect. This makes such people warm, emotional, often impulsive, and not governed too largely by logic. Ideas of the family and religion and education system are taken at face value and the thought of challenging what the father or the religious leader has said is out of the question. A lot of education would have to be shared and accepted before any Vis Dialogue could be done. Of course, there are many you may find in developing countries where this is not the case, and you can perform Holistically Counseling without trouble, perhaps even more easily than those in a more rationally-dominant society.

• **Snake Remedies/extremely loquacious**
Some people are so loquacious that they do not slow down or leave enough room for there to be a dialogue. When this occurs, I try to interrupt to get in some questions, so we can go a little deeper and not just from detail to detail of the life story. I will interrupt and say, *"One second. One second. Ok. Good. So I am hearing you tell the story now. And I feel I have enough of the story for us to now go a little deeper so I can help you. In order to do so, I'll be asking you questions that you need to consider in order to go deeper, to get to the cause of your struggles and suffering. Is that ok with you?"* Sometimes, this helps, but other times, once they begin answering a question, they are off raving again, and after several interruptions with some patients, I see that they are literally out of control with their communication, like there's a disconnect between them and the outside world, and getting questions in is out of their control. I wrote Snake Remedies, as an example of the type of patient who can be this loquacious. I had a patient who was so incredibly loquacious during our initial consultation that I could not help her with Holistic Counseling. Instead, I suggested a homeopathic snake remedy and amazingly, during our follow-up she was much less loquacious and I could actually deliver questions for her to reflect on. Nature has many gifts for us to use medicinally.

• **In control**

Some patients are just so much in control that they do not like to yield in any way. The yielding and facing the inner darkness most likely brings up a close resonance to some of their wounds, and they avoid it like the plague. The practitioner will get a sense that the patient is controlling all the answers and not in a good way, as Nature is supposed to be allowed to work therein. In such a case, a direct discussion about the situation may need to occur to point this out, or perhaps working with other modalities to soften up the situation before there is any chance of deep dialoguing.

• **Strong Miasm**

I discussed in Chapter 9 that when a miasm is encountered, it is like hitting a very dense, thick, quicksand-like feeling in the dialogue. A miasm is an inherited disease that was caused by the suppression of the external eruptions of an infectious disease and that was passed on genetically. It is also possible to get miasms in a given lifetime (for example, from the suppression of the skin eruption of an infectious illness in one's current lifetime) and not from one's ancestors, but the ancestral line is the much more frequent method of acquiring a miasm. When a miasm is encountered, it is very, very difficult to get past it. For one reason, it permeates all spaces in the person like the swamp gas it was named after (Miasma, is Greek for swamp gas). It is pervasive, insidious, and, perhaps most importantly, the patient was born with it and it is therefore believed and accepted to be inherently ingrained in their being. There is nothing to compare life to beyond the miasm, since it has been there from the start. When I encounter a miasm, I use homeopathy to assist its release. There may be other forms of medicine that help too, but I am not aware of what would help release a miasm besides giving the homeopathic nosode (the remedy prepared from the infectious disease at question) or a well-selected anti-miasmatic constitutional remedy that helps to dissolve and clear the miasm. I think it is also possible to use Holistic Counseling to clear a miasm, but it may take dozens of appointments and revisitations to the core issue of the miasm and would be a very frustrating affair; for example: the belief of not being enough, or not being good enough, or there never being enough corresponds to the psoric miasm. The belief that there is something gross or weak about me that I have to hide relates to the sycotic miasm, and the belief that there is no hope, nothing I can do, trapped, end of the line feeling lives in the syphilitic miasm. Using Holistic Counseling to get to the bottom of the core belief is like shoveling a hole in quicksand. Sure, if you shovel well enough, you'll create some space in the sand, but once you stop, it all just oozes back into place. So it is with getting to the root of a problem within a miasm.

Allegiance to another "Higher Power" or Leader

The following limitations of Holistic Counseling all share something in common. There is some strong allegiance or faithfulness that a patient has to something else, or someone else, that prevents them from trusting and opening up to The Healing Power of Nature that occurs during the Vis Dialogue.

• Strong Belief and Reliance on conventional Medicine and "Science."

This issue can lead a patient to give no credibility to the idea or thought that the mind and body are connected, or that their choices and beliefs can have any impact whatsoever on their health. It is a kind of religious thinking of conventional medicine and "science." I put science in quotation marks because it is not true science. It is somebody using the word science with their head stuck in the ground, and with very little understanding of what is true in healing. If the person is unwilling to open up to the possibility that Holism can really help them, then we are in a sort of situation of having no permission and not wanting to be there. This limitation can change. Perhaps with time, perhaps with using other modalities, it can change and the case can open up.

• **Very religious**

Holistic Counseling is a process that brings a person to face the truth about themselves. When a person is very religious, they often have the belief that truth only exists in the guise of the religious doctrine and teachings. The "go to" person for the truth is therefore the priest, rabbi, or other spiritual leader, so how can a simple healer or naturopathic doctor bring about the awareness of any sort of truth that the spiritual leader or the Holy book has not already done for them? This sort of religious dogma blocks the mind and makes it hard to do Holistic Counseling. What should be noted is that often, very religious people may be quite open initially to the Vis Dialogue, but if a limiting or false belief system is encountered that is born from the religion itself, it is almost impossible to do anything about that. And the practitioner should not even try, else they will be pushing against a mindset that is much more locked down and supported by all the followers and generations and community that are holding the same beliefs to be true. It is also possible to encounter limiting belief systems originating within the religious beliefs in a sick patient that are not directly influencing the illness. Addressing these religious beliefs will be a waste of time and the practitioner can take note of them, but not pay them any mind. But other times, a religious belief can be at the very cause of a person's disease. I published an article about this in the NDNR titled *'Holism in Auto-Immune Disease.'* In short, a Hindu woman was having tremendous issues with her husband due to both her and his religious beliefs. She was miserable and enraged at the injustice of her situation. This had led her to develop myasthenia gravis. Since she had gotten married, she was not being allowed to visit with her family much at all because, according to their beliefs, she now belonged to his family. She missed her family terribly, but could not act out against her proper role as a good Hindu wife. The case was quite amazing. I could not counsel her to change her mind, but a good remedy was revealed in the case taking. It took a long time for the situation to change for her, and I believe, it was due to the strength of the established religious beliefs that it took so long for the remedy to bring about her cure.

Full story here: http://ndnr.com/autoimmuneallergy-medicine/holism-in-autoimmune-disease/[12]

So in this case, The Healing Power of Nature could be evoked to help her, but it took a long time and it was through homeopathy that the strength of the belief was softened until she felt free enough to act and express herself in a fashion that was much more true to her heart's desire.

• Guru

The reason it is difficult to help someone who has a guru is similar to someone who has religious beliefs. They look to the guru as the source of truth, so how can you, healthcare practitioner, provide them with any sort of truth that the guru has not already done?

• New Age/Unbalanced Positive

There are a lot of teachings in the New Age world that are incredibly out of balance toward the positive. Since the most profound healing requires the facing of the negative that dwells inside of a person, having the idea that everything is happy and nice and positive can be a real block. When someone follows the movie/book *The Secret* as if it is the very truth itself, I find it difficult to have them admit and face their inner struggles. They have become somehow convinced that if they don't admit that an issue is there, then it doesn't exist. Or in other words, they believe that by paying attention to something, it becomes real. This is often taken largely out of context and grossly misunderstood, because, if a belief is already happening at the subconscious level, ignoring it only allows it to keep playing itself out without any awareness. At the time when *The Secret* was at the height of its popularity, this issue was pervasive and I had to explain the problem to people before we could continue working together, because they continued to answer such questions like this: *"Where does this problem come from?"* "Oh, there's no problem at all." *"How does it feel?"* "Great. I am so happy and healthy inside." So I would literally have to explain that healing involves facing the darkness that already lives inside of us, and becoming aware of it helps to expose it and then release it, whereas pretending it does not exist does nothing but keep it suppressed in the darkness of the subconscious mind. For some people, I'd say the majority, they understood the imbalance and with time, were able to face their inner demons and darkness. But for others, they did not want anything other than the positive in their life and we parted ways. My father once said of a woman that was very New Agey, "It's like she's so positive, she's negative." I found this extremely insightful and profound, because the positive was so overboard, there was an underlying negativity happening under the surface. Also, by facing the negative, it becomes positive. It's very good to have a positive attitude and to see things in a positive light. This, I encourage. But if one cannot go into the negative and only uses the positive as a false veneer to avoid facing their darkness, then it becomes a problem and is a limitation for Holistic Counseling. It should be noted that if a person has a great clarity of mind and can disempower a belief by not paying it any attention, then one can release the belief in this fashion without focusing on it at all. In other words, one simply "disbelieves" it. This can and does occur but requires quite a lot of clarity of mind and discipline. I found those who were very out of balance with the positive were not actually accomplishing this method in any real way, because I could sense the negativity still living beneath the surface of their conscious efforts to be positive. If the belief is not completely released, this way of "paying it no mind" can, in time, turn into an avoidance of the underlying issue if there is any doubt. In other words, a person initially is clear and says, "That belief is not real. I pay it no mind. It is not who I am." But later, they begin wrestling with the belief to "prove" to themselves that the belief is not real. At that time, the belief is holding its ground and must therefore have some seeming realness to the patient, otherwise they would not feel like they need to prove it is wrong and wrestle with it. At such a point, the darkness needs to be addressed directly. Ironic, isn't it, that by facing darkness, it disappears? And by being positive and ignoring darkness, it makes it worse? This is the very essence of the Law of Similars in homeopathy, which we see also applies to Holistic Counseling.

Chapter 37

Frequently Asked Questions

In every class, the following questions are often asked. Also, patients will sometimes bring up questions like this, so it's helpful to go over them and think of what you'd like to say in response.

Do you have an "Elevator Speech or Pitch" for Holistic Counseling?

Here is an example of an Elevator Speech for Holistic Counseling:

Holistic Counseling is a form of counseling that uses non-directional questions in a special fashion to help the practitioner connect the patient's mind with their body to establish the real root cause of illness and disease. This technique helps to empower the patient to understand how the illness in their body is a reflection of a problem in their mind. With this technique, awareness alone has been enough to heal disease in body, mind, and emotions.

Taking Responsibility for One's Health vs Being Blamed for the Illness. What is the difference?

Very often, when people are introduced to the idea that their thoughts and beliefs have manifested their illness, they have a sort of knee-jerk reaction to say, "Oh you're blaming me for my illness." It's not a very wise retort, but happens often enough nevertheless. All the practitioner needs to do is explain the difference between taking responsibility for and being empowered for their own healing versus being blamed for their illness. It is not about blaming anyone. It's about recognizing the truth that we are responsible for our illness, and since we are responsible for it, we also have the power to heal ourselves. What would you prefer: Having no say in your illness as if there is something that has simply gone wrong in your body and relying entirely on the doctor to fix you, or being responsible for both the cause and the healing of your illness?

The Big Question – What if someone is not ready?

They came to your office, didn't they? So they are ready, even if they say they are not.

That is the basic answer to this question.

If someone chose to come to your practice, you can conclude that they are, in fact, ready.

True, they may not be entirely desirous of facing their inner demons and choices that have locked down their system, mentally, emotionally, and physically. And the disease itself does gain a mind of its own with a wish to survive. So when a person says they are not ready, it is only the disease speaking or the part of them that does not wish to do what is required in order to heal. But since the practitioner has gone through their own healing and helped many others do the same, they know that the patient must face the lurking fetters of their illness. So if a person says, "I am not ready to go there." I will begin to ask them what makes them say so, and nonchalantly continue with the questioning in hopes that they get past the hurdle of inertia. If they make a very strong declaration of not being ready, then, of course, I will honor and respect that, because then it is real and not a declaration of the disease's desire to survive. And it is very, very rare that I have ever seen a patient declare, with all sincerity, that they were truly not able or willing to be ready. It has perhaps happened once or twice during the entire time I have been in practice.

What about with children? How are they making choices that have led to their illness?

Many people would ask how young children, who are before the age when they can consciously choose belief systems, manifest illness. It's a really good question and may be the #1 most frequently asked question. It's not always that simple. Here are some of the factors to consider:

One) Children often pick up and *reflect* the state of their mother (mostly) or father, while in the womb. If the mother is going through a terribly tough time, or has some deeply locked in unhealthy patterns of thought, the baby is liable to pick up on those beliefs and integrate them into their subconscious as truth. This can then lead to a disease.

Two) A child can begin believing something, i.e. making a choice of a belief, even while in the womb. I shared a case earlier in this book of a woman, who, by going deeper and deeper into her subconscious, found herself back in the womb where she recognized that, due to her disappointment in her mother, decided she would need to be co-dependent to not face her disappointment. That is a very sophisticated mental stance to adopt for a child that has yet even to be born. This early dawning of a belief system or unhealthy pattern of behavior can lead to illness.

Three) Genetic dispositions and miasms. A child can bring genetic material from the bloodline and these can manifest early on in childhood.

Four) Past lives. A child may be bringing karmic lessons from another life or past-life traumas, all rearing to go, even before they had a chance to have them triggered or experienced in any way, shape, or form in their present life.

Five) We choose our parents. This is a very spiritual/esoteric thought to consider. Even if a child may not consciously be aware of how or why they have manifested their illness, they did choose, on some level of the soul, to come to this life and choose their parents, with all their baggage, wounds, and illness. It may be for their own growth that they chose their parents or for an important life lesson for their parents. I tell a story in class that I heard from Barry Neil Kauffman that is always a real tear-jerker whenever I tell it. The story illustrates how a child would not let go of their disease until the mother was ready to let go of the fear and control surrounding her daughter's disease.

Whatever may be the reason or cause behind a child's illness, if they are very young, you won't be able to use Holistic Counseling anyway to help them. Homeopathy or other modalities may be necessary to help the child. And treating the affected parent is of equal importance and at times, all that needs to be done in order to help a child. If a very controlling, negative parent is at the cause of the child's illness, and they are unwilling to undergo treatment, it is a bleak situation for that child. One can do all they can, but if the practitioner is only bailing out a sinking boat, it becomes futile. Perhaps trying to keep the boat afloat to the greatest degree and for as long as possible, is all we can do at times to alleviate suffering.

Use of supplements? Vitamins?

Giving supplements or vitamins that support the body nutritionally are fine. This can work in harmony with Holism. Giving supplements that have many medically active ingredients and herbs that are created specifically for a condition or disease, in my opinion, is not good. They, like drugs, are designed to treat the symptoms of disease and thus create suppression, worsening the Vital Force due to the blockage of the expression of the symptoms, and thus, in the end, they are doing some harm. I would recommend these to be stopped and often do so, in order to help a patient recover fully and not depend on the supplements as a crutch. It is the same as with drugs. Supplements and herbal preparations act as drugs when they are administered specifically for conditions and symptoms. Sure, they are more natural, but they still act in the same model as their pharmaceutical allopathic counterparts.

Holsitic Counseling is a lot like Homeopathy. They both are very subtle medicines. They both endeavor to target the pathology by it being faced, both in their own way. And, both can be upset or offset by intervening factors that throw the remedy or the holism off the tracks. In the Organon, Hahnemann states: "Due to the necessary, as well as the expedient, minuteness of the dose used in the homeopathic procedure, it is easy to grasp why, during treatment, everything else that could, in any way, act medicinally, must be removed from the diet and regimen, so that the subtle dose will not be overtuned and extinguished or even disturbed by any foreign medicinal irritant."[21]

I have described many situations where the drugs did block the treatment and needed to be removed. The same was the case for the supplements. Sometimes it is due to the fact that the supplements are the outside helpers, the mythological supporters in the patient's mind, so that they do not have to take responsibility and change their way of thinking nor their way of life. In such cases, the supplements act quite contrary to the direction of healing and must be removed. Other times the patient is just taking too many in a desperate attempt to throw whatever they can at the disease, and are overwhelming their liver and their kidneys in an attempt to digest all the supplements (not to mention their pocket books). Or they have been prescribed all these supplements by naturopaths, chiropractors and other alternative healthcare practitioners to allopathically address each issue that a patient has. This is the very worse way of practicing Naturopathic medicine and is the main reason that naturopaths have become notorious as supplement pushers. It's also a questionable conflict of interest when naturopaths have their own dispensaries and make a lot of profit from selling supplements. Sure, not every naturopath that has a dispensary is motivated by money and only has the supplements there as a convenience for their patients. Someone has to make money off the supplements, might as well be the practitioner. That is fine. But there is no reason that a patient should leave with hundreds of dollars of supplements.

The following are examples of good and bad forms of nutritional supplementation within the context of working holistically and in harmony with Holistic Counseling. None of these treatments are bad, per se, but this comparison is to look at where it could mean moving the patient in opposite directions – holistic, root-cause, whole person, or suppression of symptoms allopathically.

Examples of good nutritional support – Giving maternity vitamins for pregnant women. Giving Vitamin D, calcium, magnesium, and phosphates for a child that often fractures their bones while working holistically to improve the disposition toward injury. Giving manganese to support the immune system for someone with myasthenia gravis while they work on the root cause of their illness. Putting skin nourishing oils, creams, and soothing herbs like Vitamin E, coconut oil, and calendula on the skin to soothe and ease the skin. Nutritional changes that are applied through the diet are always welcome, as well as telling patients to avoid certain inflammatory foods or foods that exacerbate their condition, like sugar, wheat, dairy, soy, etc. and where a person can gain the nutrients they need via the diet is always preferable to giving a nutritional supplement or vitamin. Also, detoxification and cleansing protocols can be helpful and harmonious during holistic healing. This is not an exhaustive list. It's just some examples to illustrate that nutritional support of the body is ok while working in chronic illness. Working in acute cases of disease is different and may involve more symptomatic targeted approach, depending on the severity of the illness and the situation.

Examples of bad nutritional support – Giving an immune modulator for an auto-immune disease.
Giving a supplement with many herbs and/or other medicinally active ingredients for a particular condition, e.g., hypothyroidism, constipation, depression, anxiety, insomnia, low back

pain.

Topical creams with active medicinal ingredients for skin conditions. Giving anxiolytic herbs or supplements for anxiety. Giving antidepressants for depression. Giving nervines and "sleeping supplements" for insomnia. Basically anything that says, "Take this supplement for this condition."

Gray Zone – Sometimes, a patient is very fed up and needs a little relief before continuing with the deep stuff. Or they are exhausted and need some support. Adrenal support may be indicated in such a case so that the patient does not worsen during their exhaustion. Also, at times, a patient is overwhelmed by life, working at a demanding job or jobs, taking care of the kids, and trying to deal with their health. Or a patient has undergone some tremendous trauma or shock and just needs to have some reprieve from their grief or anxiety. At such times, sometimes they do need a crutch to get through. They are in that gray zone where they are not really able to deal with their illness at the root cause anyway, so we might as well help support them. I do not find the need to treat this way very often. But it does happen from time to time. And I often do use homeopathy instead of herbal medicine or supplements to do so, but once we're applying an allopathic support or temporary fix, whatever does the trick is good, so long as it doesn't cause harmful toxicity and side effects. In very aggressive cases of cancer, a multifold approach is needed that definitely works directly on targeting the tumor and works to help organs of digestion and elimination. There are also some conditions, like LYME disease, that require direct targeting of a chronic infection to help bring about healing, along with the mind-body approach.

In any given case, the choice of how to apply supplements is at the discretion of the practitioner. In a certain case, if the practitioner recognizes that they are giving too many supplements and it is interfering with their patient's desire to make changes to their belief systems, then they will learn from that mistake. In other cases, it will become clear that a little support while the patient makes a difficult transition is appropriate. A practitioner that wishes to become proficient in holistic healing in general and specifically Holistic Counseling should not give supplements to treat the symptoms just because they are not getting the results they desire, lest they never improve past the point they are getting stuck with their patients. Rather, a practitioner should instead look inside of themselves for the reason they are getting stuck with their patients, and endeavor to heal and grow in the way necessary to improve as a practitioner.

What about if you give a homeopathic and do Holistic Counseling and the patient improves – how do you know what did what?

This is a good question and one that is worthy of consideration. The first answer, which is spoken by me the Naturopathic doctor and healer, is that it doesn't matter what did what, as long as the patient is improving. The ultimate goal is to ensure that a patient improves, so what does it matter? But that is not really a satisfactory answer from the scientific homeopathic and Holistic Counseling perspectives. Sometimes, it is difficult to tell what did what, and so, you may need to repeat the whole process in order to continue with the improvements. I have noticed, however, that patients do seem to have a sense of what improved them and what did not. They will sometimes tell me that they noticed immediate benefits following our Holistic Counseling session and they haven't seen any improvements just with the remedy. At times, I get this sense too and do agree. Not to make matters more complicated, but homeopathy is so often and so easily dismissed by patients that I don't always believe them when they say that the remedy hasn't worked. I will go through their symptoms, and in particular, their SRPs (Strange, Rare and Peculiar symptoms) and if I notice that many aspects of their body, emotions, and mind have improved, it is hard to attribute that strictly to the Holistic Counseling. For example, a person has a shift in their belief that they alone are responsible for everyone in their family, and that improves their life, but many of the other symptoms, like dreams, constipation, insomnia, shortness of breath, food cravings, and other physical or general symptoms do not change with the remedy. This is a sign that the remedy did not act very deeply and is likely not the right remedy, provided enough time has elapsed to give it a fair trial. It is possible that a person has a constitutional shift from a change in their fundamental core belief system, but as a practitioner gets experienced using homeopathy and Holistic Counseling, they will be able to discern more easily what is doing what in the case. There are times when I do notice a change in the patient and then during the next follow-up it is clear that the changes from the Holistic Counseling have held, but not much else has improved. This is a sign that the remedy is not right or is not acting and the Holistic Counseling, alone, did help. Other times, a patient didn't have much of a shift during the dialogue, but after they begin their remedy everything improves. This is a clear sign that the homeopathy did the trick and the Holistic Counseling did not or, it just did a little loosening up before the remedy did the majority of the healing.

In certain cases, if we are unable to determine what did what, does it really matter? Though I honor and highly respect homeopathy, I am not so much of a purist that I will not conduct Holistic Counseling at the same time. They both work in the same fashion – in harmony with The Healing Power of Nature. And as I shared in Chapter 9, *The Vital Force – Implications for Holistic Counseling*, I explained how Hahnemann's views of counseling were of the practitioner providing "displays of trust, friendly exhortations, reasoning with the patient, and even well-camouflaged deception."[11] I believe it is for this reason that homeopaths have had a bias against mixing counseling and homeopathy. In a true Holistic Counseling session, we do not input our own awareness, nor provide displays of trust, friendly exhortations or reasoning with the patient. We, ideally, are working quite in harmony with homeopathy and so the two do work very well together toward the same goal – the healing of the patient.

When I used to work strictly as a homeopath, I was relying entirely on my skills as a homeopath to get results. At times, I was unable to get a good, deep acting remedy for four or five appointments. That means four or five paid appointments where a patient has essentially not benefitted from seeing me at all. Yes, when the *Similimum* is found, there is little that compares to homeopathy, but what about when we are unable to find it for some time? I have seen quite a few patients not return when I relied solely on homeopathy. And can I blame them for not returning when I had selected remedies that were not acting? However, when a patient says, "Good question!" and you got them thinking deeply and introspectively, and you have helped change their life forever by your simple, open-ended, non-directional questions following the stream, then they know how valuable the appointments are and they will return for more healing.

Can I do Holistic Counseling on close family and friends?

The answer is: You can do it with loved ones, but you have to be able to harness great detachment and not get involved in trying to fix them. I have counseled close people in my family and I was able to help them a lot. Sometimes I do get too involved, but overall, I can be helpful for them when I am as detached as possible.

Can you harness detachment? For those people where you feel it would be really hard to detach, and especially where you are involved, the most likely best bet is to refer to someone else. If not, it can get messy and cause a schism in the relationship. I've noticed that it did change the dynamic with some friends that I have Holistically Counseled. And that makes sense. So that is another consideration.

It really depends on the person – some can handle it and be vulnerable and also still be friends.

For others, they feel they have "lost" something in the connection, and then it's hard to get back the innocence of just the friendship.

Can I do Holistic Counseling on myself?

Yes. It is best to write down each of the questions and answers. Or type them all up. Otherwise, you can get lost in the sequence of things and will find it hard to proceed with further questions. One must also be very detached and unbiased. It may sound like a challenge, and it is, but it is still possible to do this and get good results. However, it is preferable, as with any form of healing, to interact with another person. Just as it is possible to acupuncture oneself, (except perhaps on certain points on the back) the exchange of someone else needling you makes a big difference as there is an exchange of energy and not a closed system. That analogy, however, works only in part when exploring working on oneself with Holistic Counseling, because if one is able to get to the core, change the belief and be released, on one's own, it is pretty much the same as doing it with another. The thing is that another person provides insights and good feedback and directions with the questions that we may not think of ourselves. That is the great advantage of having outside help.

With time, as one gets good at moving through the layers of their rabbit hole and their beliefs, it becomes possible to ask one question, such as, *"What am I feeling right now?"* and to follow a very fast chain of responses and subsequent questions right down to the root of the problem in any given moment. As we become accustomed to this process of looking within and learning about ourselves, awareness can arrive in a flash, where we can immediately detect what is bothering us when we begin to feel uncomfortable or upset about a given situation or event and ask, *"What is this about?"*

Holistic Counseling – In Conclusion

There you have it. All you need to go and tackle the toughest cases with simple, effective questions. By studying this book and getting acquainted with the different elements of it, you will be able to recognize in a given case where you are, and where you need to go to help someone. You will not feel lost or as if you are flailing. Remember, this book is meant as a supplement to part 1 and part 2 of Holistic Counseling – The Course, and is not meant as a stand-alone teaching instrument, as there are crucial elements learned from a live course that one cannot gather from a book alone. Initially, to make the transition between the static, "neat and clean" form of the book into the sometimes messy, dynamic, drawn-out, and unpredictable form of the live case; take your time and just follow the stream. You may feel lost and unsure of what to ask at a certain point. If so, you can give some feedback to "buy time." You can allow for a breathing space, for things to bubble to the surface, either by you, the practitioner, or the patient. You can even have a list of the questions and choose one that pops to the surface. Follow your gut, your instinct. Holistic Counseling is forgiving and allows for error. There is room for poor questions, and incorrect feedback, because the patient is always there to correct the mistakes of the practitioner and to bring more clarity to the matter at hand. And some cases are so uniquely troubled and challenging, that only the most creatively spun, off-the-cuff, ad-libbed questions will result in an opening and progress.

If you find yourself hesitating or tripping up at the same situations in more than one case, it is time to examine what that sort of a situation brings up for your own "Physician, Heal Thyself!" Is it a fear of challenging a patient's resistance to facing their issues? What makes that difficult for you? Are you having a hard time asking non-directional questions when a patient is close to seeing the answer for themselves? What makes you need to jump in at such a point in the dialogue? Is it difficult for you to "close the deal?" If so, you can go over the reading, review the various approaches and techniques, to see if you were missing something. And if not, what keeps getting in the way about "closing the deal?"

If you're still struggling in a certain aspect of the practice and cannot seem to find a solution, then bring your issue to the Forum and we will try to help you resolve it. There is also an extensive resource of practitioners who have learned the technique that you can partner up with to do exchanges of Holistic Counseling sessions to help you improve your technique and continue to heal yourself.

What you have at your fingertips is a profound and effective method for healing. How much you use it is entirely up to you. Most students that take the course recognize the validity and importance of it. Yet how much they really apply it in practice is most certainly a reflection of how much they are applying it upon themselves. This is why "Physician, Heal Thyself!" remains one of the most important factors in holistic practice. It is clear that practitioners practice very much in relation to what they use on themselves. A seasoned homeopath receives a scare with cancer, and decides to undergo chemo and radiation treatment. Subsequently, their attitude and philosophy change toward medicine and they become more evidence-based and allopathic as a reflection of their decisions for their own health. I've seen students really be inspired in the course that do not apply the method in practice because they have not taken it home enough. What you walk, you talk and practice. If you don't want to "go there" for your own healing, why and how would you ever bring another there in practice?

The path is a committed one. To be or not to be is the question of being aligned with one's I AM statement. The same is true for the commitment to walking a path devoted to true holistic healing. It may be hard. It may be painful. It may even be frightening. But it's worth it. Every ounce of struggle and pain is worth it, because there will always be breakthroughs, even through the most challenging of issues. And when one breaks through to a deeper level, being healthier, more vibrant, and more alive is reward enough.

I want to express my sincere gratitude that you have taken your time to read this entire book. I extend to you my even greater appreciation if you are among the ranks of those who have chosen to embrace the Holistic path of Naturopathic medicine, of medicine in general, and of healing and that you practice Holistic Counseling – The Vis Dialogue. And the world thanks you, as the doctors who could really help people heal at the deepest part of their illness have been few in number, and now, thanks to you, there are more of us. In time, it is my hope to see a great change in the way people regard medicine as a whole, and that the beautiful, holistic and vitality-based medicine of Naturopathy will reclaim its principles and align with its roots, so it can be much more impactful and truly healing to the world.

May the Healing Power of Nature be ever guiding you towards greater personal health and well-being and may you continue to experience the honor and the joy of helping change people's health and lives for the better.

From Dr. Moshe

Thank you so much for reading *Holistic Counseling – Introducing "The Vis Dialogue."* My sincere hope is that the model of Holism has been edified enough in your own mind that you will be able to bring it forward to help many people with it. In the spirit of helping others benefit from this wholesome model of healing and from the book, if you have a few moments, would you please add your review of the book at your favorite online site for feedback?

(Amazon, Apple iTunes Store, GoodReads, etc.)

Also, if you would like to connect with others and get updates on the up and coming events we'll be holding, please Like Us on Facebook at: www.facebook.com/holisticcounselingcourse

Sincerely,
Dr. Moshe Daniel Block, ND

Appendix

About the Course and Certification

In order to be certified, a practitioner must take Part 1, Part 2 of the Holistic Counseling class, and then do the final Certification process.

For Part 1; Anyone is eligible to take part 1, though I much prefer to offer these profound healing techniques to healthcare practitioners that will be applying the knowledge to heal themselves and their patients/clients. Knowledge in medicine, homeopathy and other modalities of medicine is helpful for the course, though not required.

Following Part 1, a student must practice on 10 patients (can be friends and family as practice) and then write up 2 cases with the Holistic Counseling Vis Dialogue Self-Assessment form.

Here are the criteria for the write ups: These have to be submitted no later than 1 week before the Part 2 class.

And note: Even though only 2 written up cases are required, a student should/could use this self-assessment to monitor their progress & growth for each and every case taken. It is remarkable how helpful and insightful these self-assessments are for students as they practice the Dialogue.

Holistic Counseling Vis Dialogue Self-Assessment:

1) How did you feel doing the dialogue?

A) What did you feel comfortable with?

B) What did you feel uncomfortable with?

C) Please list some of your favorite and/or most-natural questions during the dialogue.

D) What is most difficult about the Vis Dialogue for you? How does this relate to where you need to "Physician, Heal Thyself?"

2) Were you able to be "non-directional?" if so, share your experience of it.

Were you controlling/directing the dialogue too much?

If so,can you detect what need/issue inside of yourself led you to do so?

Were there any issues that came up that triggered you? If so, what were they and where does that come from for you personally?

3) How balanced were you with your male-female energies? Did you tend to be too male or too female? How did this impact your practice?

4) A) Did your patient have any breakthroughs?

B) What underlying core beliefs did you help your patient discover?

C) What minor beliefs/patterns did you help your patient discover?

5) Were you able to "close" the appointment to help the patient discover the choice and implement it for change? If so, please describe which techniques/questions you used to do so?

If you had trouble, please describe what you struggled with to help them make the choice and let go.

6) A) Are you a member of the Forums or Holistic Counseling?

http://www.holistic-counseling.ca/Forums/

B) Please feel free to write any thoughts, comments, or questions about the process either here or in a new thread on the Forums.

Note: A student should not submit the notes from the write-ups of the cases. Just the self-assessment questions are enough.

For Part 2: a student understands that by taking Part 2 of Holistic Counseling, you agree not to teach this technique to anyone. If you wish to become an instructor in Holistic Counseling, there will be an opportunity in the future to take a teacher's training class. This will be available to practitioners that have taken Part 1, Part 2, done the Certification process, and have practiced for a minimum of three years, demonstrating excellence in the Vis Dialogue.

By taking Part 2 of Holistic Counseling, you also understand that Part 2 is the last class before a practitioner of Holistic Counseling can become certified in Holistic Counseling. Following part 2, a student will practice a minimum of 15 cases before taking the final step for Certification. There is a final step before the Certification process is complete that involves recording videos of two cases of 1 hour each, and submitting these videos to Dr. Moshe for assessment. The assessment for Certification costs $350 US (this fee may be subject to change). Once certified, you can advertise on your website and in your office/practice that you are a certified Holistic Counselor, being proficient in the Vis Dialogue. You will also have a small bio listed on the official Holistic Counseling website stating that you are certified in the Vis Dialogue. Referral programs will be available to interested practitioners. Before that time, you may tell patients and people who you practice on that you have learned Holistic Counseling – The Vis Dialogue, but are not yet certified. Before Certification, you may not advertise on your website or marketing material that you do Holistic Counseling.

References

1. Schucman H. The Separation and the Atonement. In: *A Course In Miracles*. 1st ed. Mill Valley: Foundation for Inner Peace; 2007:23.
2. Schucman H. The Separation and the Atonement. In: *A Course In Miracles*. 1st ed. Mill Valley: Foundation for Inner Peace; 2007:24.
3. Pathwaysoflight.org. A Course in Miracles Text Q&A on Chapter 2: The Separation and the Atonement, Section IV: Healing as Release from Fear. 2015. Available at: http://www.pathwaysoflight.org/%20acim_text/answers/sec tion_iv_healing_as_release_from_fear. Accessed July 13, 2015.
4. Hamilton G, Wheeler P. *The Golden Chain Of Homer*. 1st ed. Bloomington: iUniverse; 2012.
5. Hamilton G, Wheeler P. *The Golden Chain Of Homer*. 1st ed. Bloomington: iUniverse; 2012:37.
6. Davis P. Introducing the Bio-Energetic Work of Wilhelm Reich. *Orgone Therapy*. Available at: http://www.orgone therapy.biz/. Accessed July 13, 2015.
7. Brennan B. *Hands Of Light*. Toronto: Bantam Books; 1988:45.
8. Brennan B. *Light Emerging*. New york: Bantam Books; 1993:265.
9. Holistic. *Oxford Dictionaries*. 2015. Available at: http://www.oxforddictionaries.com/definition/english/holist ic. Accessed July 13, 2015.
10 Hahnemann S, O'Reilly W. *Organon Of The Medical Art*. Redmond, Wash.: Birdcage Books; 1996:65.
11. Hahnemann S, O'Reilly W. *Organon Of The Medical Art*. Redmond, Wash.: Birdcage Books; 1996:202-203.
12. Block M. Holism in Autoimmune Disease. *NDNR*. 2015. Available at: http://ndnr.com/autoimmuneallergy-medi

cine/holism-in-autoimmune-disease/. Accessed July 13, 2015.

13. Pond D. *Universal Laws Never Before Revealed: Keely's Secrets*. Santa Fe, NM: Message Co.; 1995.

14. Hay L. *You Can Heal Your Life*. Santa Monica, CA: Hay House; 1987.

15. Nondirective. *Merriam-Webster*. 2015. Available at: http://www.merriam-webster.com/dictionary/nondirective. Accessed July 13, 2015.

16. *Seven Years In Tibet*. Tibet, China; La Plata, Buenos Aires; Mendoza, Argentina: Jean-Jacques Annaud; 1997.

17. Epstein P. Where's the Healing? *NDNR*. 2007. Available at: http://ndnr.com/mindbody/wheres-the-healing/. Accessed July 13, 2015.

18. Block M. Managing Mind Body Medicine in a World of Obstacles. *NDNR*. 2013. Available at: http://ndnr.com/mindbody/managing-mind-body-medicine-in-a-world-of-obstacles/. Accessed July 13, 2015.

19. Jung C. *Memories, Dreams, Reflections*. New York: Pantheon Books; 1963.

20. Block M. *The Last Four Books Of Moses*. Montreal, Quebec, Canada: Collective Co-op Pub.; 2004:90.

21. Hahnemann S, O'Reilly W. *Organon Of The Medical Art*. Redmond, Wash.: Birdcage Books; 1996:227.

**PSYCHE
BOOKS**

The study of the mind: interactions, behaviours, functions.
Developing and learning our understanding of self. Psyche
Books cover all aspects of psychology and matters relating to
the head.

Printed and bound by CPI Group (UK) Ltd, Croydon, CR0 4YY

12/05/2025

01867612-0005